DOSAGE CALCULATIONS
IN SI UNITS

Third Edition

DOSAGE CALCULATIONS IN SI UNITS

MAUREEN OSIS, R.N., M.N.

Clinical Nurse Specialist, Geriatrics
Calgary District Hospital Group
Adjunct Assistant Professor, Faculty of Nursing,
University of Calgary

THIRD EDITION

with 125 illustrations

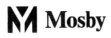 **Mosby**

St. Louis   Baltimore   Berlin   Boston   Carlsbad   Chicago   London   Madrid
Naples   New York   Philadelphia   Sydney   Tokyo   Toronto

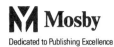
Dedicated to Publishing Excellence

Publisher: Alison Harrison
Managing Editor: Jeff Burnham
Associate Developmental Editor: Linda Caldwell
Project Manager: Barbara Bowles Merritt
Designer: David Zielinski
Manufacturing Supervisor: Betty Richmond
Cover Art: Catherine Chang

3rd EDITION
Copyright © by Mosby-Year Book, Inc.

Previous editions copyrighted 1986, 1991

A NOTE TO THE READER
The author and publisher have made every attempt to check dosages and nursing content for accuracy. Because the science of pharmacology is continually advancing, the knowledge base continues to expand. Therefore, we recommend that the reader always check product information for changes in dosage or administration before administering any medication. This is particularly important with new or rarely used drugs.

Printed in Canada
Composition by Page Two Associates, Inc.
Printing/binding by Bryant Press

Mosby-Year Book, Inc.
11830 Westline Industrial Drive, St. Louis, Missouri 63146

Library of Congress Cataloging in Publication Data

Osis, M. (Maureen)
  Dosage calculation in SI units

3rd ed.
ISBN 0-8151-6549-8

1. Drugs — Dosage.   2. Pharmaceutical arithmetic.
I. Title.

    95 96 97 / 9 8 7 6 5 4 3 2 1

Dedication

In loving memory of Dad

PREFACE

The first edition of *Dosage Calculations in SI Units* in 1986, began with a quote from Florence Nightingale. She wrote;

> "I have known several of our real old-fashioned sisters, who could as accurately as a measuring glass, measure out all their patients' wine and medicine by the eye, and never be wrong. I do not recommend this, one must be very sure of one's self to do it."
>
> Florence Nightingale, Notes on Nursing, 1859

I return to this quote because the phrase of being "very sure of one's self" applies more than ever in today's complex health care settings. This edition is written for nurses, nursing students, and other health care providers who must accurately calculate doses, both simple and complex, in a variety of settings. The book is an investment in safe clinical practice because it provides the basic knowledge required for calculation and many exercises and simulations to develop competence and confidence.

Important Features

- takes the learner from simple and familiar to more complex skills
- recognizes that readers will differ in basic knowledge and ability and organizes the content accordingly
- provide simulations of the demands of the real clinical setting (i.e., case studies, and actual medication labels)
- offers many exercises so the learner can master one skill before proceeding to the next

How to Use this Book

to the nursing instructor

As with the previous editions, you may wish to assign use of the book independently or as an adjunct to classroom, laboratory, and clinical learning. The book should not be used entirely in one term; for example, modules 1–6 could be completed in conjunction with laboratory demonstrations on medication administration, whereas module 7 should be completed in conjunction with intravenous certification. Modules 8 and 9 provide more complex and specialized information that will be relevant to the more advanced nursing student.

This edition retains a sample examination for your use in the Appendix. A CAI program is available for purchase and can be used on IBM computers.

to other instructors

This book is also useful for other health care providers. For example, licensed practical nurses will find Modules 1–5 useful to provide the foundation for oral administration. The content was reviewed by a pharmacist to ensure that it is also appropriate for the pharmacy technicians.

to the student

This book assumes that you have basic arithmetic skills and offers only a brief review of the arithmetic of whole numbers, fractions, and decimal numbers. If you do not achieve 100% in Module 1, you will require additional remedial assistance. You should proceed through the modules in sequence and be certain you are competent using ratio and proportion before attempting calculations. Develop a habit for safe practice - always check your answers intuitively (does it make sense?) and then validate the answer using the equation statement.

Acknowledgements

I wish to thank the following companies for allowing me to reproduce medication labels:
Adria Laboratories, Columbus, Ohio
Bristol Laboratories, Princeton, New Jersey
Bristol-Myers Squibb Canada, Inc., Montreal, Quebec
Burroughs Wellcome, Research Triangle Park, North Carolina
Eli Lilly Canada Inc., Scarborough, Ontario
Eli Lilly and Company, Indianapolis, Indiana
Elkins-Sinn Inc., Cherry Hill, New Jersey
Geigy Pharmaceuticals, Ardsley, New York
Hoechst-Roussel Pharmaceuticals Inc., Somerville, New Jersey
Lederle Laboratories, Pearl River, New York
Leo Laboratories Canada Inc., Ajax, Ontario
Mead Johnson Pharmaceuticals, Evansville, Indiana
Novo Nordisk Canada Inc., Mississauga, Ontario
Parke-Davis, Morris Plains, New Jersey
Roerig, New York, New York
Roxane Laboratories Inc., Columbus, Ohio
Schering Corporation, Kenilworth, New Jersey
SmithKline Beecham Pharma Inc., Oakville, Ontario
The Upjohn Company, Kalamazoo, Michigan
Wyeth-Ayerst Laboratories, Philadelphia, Pennsylvania

and

Manrex Limited, Winnipeg, Manitoba for allowing me to reproduce various types of medication delivery systems.

Many individuals reviewed the second edition and provided valuable suggestions for this book. Wherever possible, I have tried to incorporate these suggestions in the third edition. In particular I would like to thank the following individuals:

- Martha Nystrom, B.S.P., M.B.A. for her thorough critique of the exercises and her precise definitions of concepts and terms

- Sheena Mainland for sharing her expertise as a pediatric nurse clinician and writing several exercises.

- Carol Straub and Carrol Morris, nursing instructors at Wascana Institute, Regina, Saskatchewan, for their thoughtful reviews of math calculations and content.

- John Martel, Professor of Health and Biology at St. Clair College of Applied Arts and Technology, Windsor, Ontario, for an extremely helpful review that supported the strengths of the previous edition while identifying opportunities for improvement.

- Gladys Rangaratnam, Professor, Cambrian College of Applied Arts and Technology, Sudbury, Ontario, for reviewing math calculations to ensure accuracy.

My thanks to Linda Caldwell, Associate Developmental Editor of the Nursing Division, for her patience and perseverance in taking this edition from idea to reality.

I cannot close without again thanking my family, Imants, Andrew, Lara, and Sean, for carrying the load while I spent hours on the computer!

Maureen Osis

Brief Contents

Detailed Contents

Module 1: Arithmetic of Whole Numbers, Fractions, and Decimal Numbers

This module provides a self-check and brief review of basic arithmetic skills of whole numbers, fractions and decimal numbers. You should complete the pretest to assess your skills. If you do not achieve 100%, assess your areas of weakness and complete some or all of the brief review in the module. Write the posttest. If you do not achieve 100%, you should seek remedial assistance, which is beyond the scope of this book.

PRETEST

Instructions

1. Write the test without referring to any resources.
2. Correct the test using the answer guide.
3. If your score is 100%, proceed to module 2.
4. If you do not achieve 100%, proceed through the module topics, then write the posttest.

Part I. Arithmetic of Whole Numbers

1.
$$\begin{array}{r} 546 \\ +\ 677 \\ \hline 1223 \end{array}$$

2.
$$\begin{array}{r} 1\ 972 \\ +\ 545 \\ \hline 2517 \end{array}$$

3.
$$\begin{array}{r} 729 \\ +\ 85 \\ \hline 814 \end{array}$$

4.
$$\begin{array}{r} 139 \\ +\ 455 \\ \hline 594 \end{array}$$

5.
$$\begin{array}{r} 831 \\ -\ 356 \\ \hline 475 \end{array}$$

6.
$$\begin{array}{r} 1\ 897 \\ -\ 543 \\ \hline 1354 \end{array}$$

7.
$$\begin{array}{r} 3\ 452 \\ -\ 399 \\ \hline 53 \end{array}$$

8.
$$\begin{array}{r} 894 \\ -\ 105 \\ \hline 789 \end{array}$$

9.
$$\begin{array}{r} 876 \\ \times\ 59 \\ \hline 51684 \end{array}$$

10.
$$\begin{array}{r} 645 \\ \times\ 13 \\ \hline 8385 \end{array}$$

11.
$$\begin{array}{r} 3\ 789 \\ \times\ 235 \end{array}$$

12.
$$\begin{array}{r} 1\ 094 \\ \times\ 2001 \end{array}$$

13. $11\overline{)55}$ 5

14. $12\overline{)96}$

15. $25\overline{)125}$

Part I: Your Score: _____ /15 = _____ %

Note: The Metric Commission of Canada states that spaces are used to separate long numbers into three-digit blocks e.g., 123 456. With four-digit numbers, the space is optional, e.g., 1 972 or 1972.

Part II. Arithmetic of Fractions (simplify if necessary)

1. $\dfrac{3}{9} + \dfrac{7}{13} =$

2. $\dfrac{5}{7} + \dfrac{3}{16} =$

3. $\dfrac{1}{6} + \dfrac{3}{5} =$

4. $\dfrac{11}{12} + \dfrac{1}{2} =$

5. $\dfrac{2}{5} + 3\dfrac{1}{4} =$

6. $\dfrac{1}{3} + \dfrac{7}{10} + \dfrac{1}{5} =$

7. $2 + \dfrac{3}{4} =$

8. $3\dfrac{1}{8} + 4\dfrac{1}{6} =$

9. $\dfrac{3}{4} - \dfrac{5}{16} =$

10. $\dfrac{11}{12} - \dfrac{2}{3} =$

11. $\dfrac{19}{24} - \dfrac{1}{2} =$

12. $\dfrac{7}{8} - \dfrac{5}{6} =$

13. $\dfrac{7}{8} - \dfrac{2}{9} =$

14. $1\dfrac{1}{4} - \dfrac{3}{5} =$

15. $3 - \dfrac{7}{16} =$

16. $9\dfrac{3}{8} - 6\dfrac{7}{16} =$

17. $4\dfrac{7}{8} \times 5\dfrac{6}{7} =$

18. $2\dfrac{5}{6} \times \dfrac{1}{2} =$

19. $\dfrac{3}{4} \times 9\dfrac{15}{16} =$

20. $3\dfrac{1}{3} \times 2\dfrac{1}{2} =$

21. $\dfrac{2}{3} \times \dfrac{3}{4} =$

22. $3\dfrac{1}{4} \times 4\dfrac{1}{2} =$

23. $16 \times \dfrac{3}{10} =$

24. $3\dfrac{1}{2} \times 9 =$

25. $\dfrac{7}{8} \div \dfrac{3}{5} =$

26. $\dfrac{9}{16} \div \dfrac{3}{4} =$

27. $3\dfrac{1}{4} \div \dfrac{1}{3} =$

28. $\dfrac{5}{9} \div \dfrac{7}{10} =$

29. $\dfrac{16}{27} \div \dfrac{2}{3} =$

31. $76 \div \dfrac{3}{4} =$

30. $1\dfrac{1}{2} \div \dfrac{1}{2} =$

32. $\dfrac{9}{16} \div 3 =$

Change These Improper Fractions to Mixed or Whole Numbers

33. $\dfrac{18}{5} =$

36. $\dfrac{127}{34} =$

34. $\dfrac{83}{11} =$

37. $\dfrac{39}{8} =$

35. $\dfrac{49}{6} =$

38. $\dfrac{125}{12} =$

Find the Lowest Common Denominator

39. $\dfrac{1}{2}$ and $\dfrac{1}{4}$

41. $\dfrac{5}{8}$ and $\dfrac{2}{5}$

40. $\dfrac{1}{5}$ and $\dfrac{1}{6}$

42. $\dfrac{2}{3}$ and $\dfrac{7}{8}$

Simplify These Fractions to Their Lowest Terms

43. $\dfrac{21}{24} =$

46. $\dfrac{15}{35} =$

44. $\dfrac{18}{72} =$

47. $\dfrac{20}{32} =$

45. $\dfrac{6}{9} =$

48. $\dfrac{5}{75} =$

Identify the Following Expressions as Proper or Improper Fractions or Mixed Numbers

49. $\dfrac{7}{15}$

51. $1\dfrac{7}{8}$

50. $\dfrac{21}{11}$

52. $\dfrac{1}{30}$

53. $\dfrac{1}{17}$

55. $3\dfrac{1}{10}$

54. $\dfrac{6}{7}$

56. $\dfrac{9}{5}$

Equivalent Fractions

Express each fraction as an equivalent fraction.

57. $\dfrac{1}{2} = \dfrac{?}{6}$

60. $\dfrac{7}{10} = \dfrac{49}{?}$

58. $\dfrac{3}{20} = \dfrac{9}{?}$

61. $\dfrac{1}{5} = \dfrac{6}{?}$

59. $\dfrac{7}{9} = \dfrac{?}{27}$

Are the following expressions equivalent fractions?

62. $\dfrac{3}{8} = \dfrac{15}{30}$ Yes or No

63. $\dfrac{21}{30} = \dfrac{126}{180}$ Yes or No

Change to Improper Fractions

64. $6\dfrac{1}{8} =$

65. $7\dfrac{9}{10} =$

66. $5\dfrac{1}{2} =$

For each of the following pairs, choose the correct way of writing decimals. Circle your choice.

67.   .25 or 0.25

69.   0.120 or 0.12

68.   1.0 or 1

70.   .5 or 0.5

Part II: Your Score: _____ /70 = _____ %

Part III. Arithmetic of Decimal Numbers

1. Write "one-half" in correct decimal format.

Rounding Decimal Numbers

Round the following decimal numbers to the nearest tenth.

2. 3.43   4. 1.239

3. 7.09   5. 9.16

Round the following decimal numbers to the nearest hundredth.

6. 12.459   8. 34.007

7. 6.086   9. 4.909

Addition of Decimal Numbers

10. $1.567 + 0.98 =$ 12. $0.4 + 5.6 + 0.27 =$

11. $123.5 + 2.534\ 2 =$ 13. $2.1 + 0.53 + 1.102 =$

Subtraction of Decimal Numbers

14. $10 - 3.7 =$ 16. $5.6 - 1.08 =$

15. $4.2 - 0.9 =$ 17. $0.125 - 0.075 =$

Multiplication of Decimal Numbers

18. $0.8 \times 10 =$ 20. $0.8 \times 1\ 000 =$

19. $0.8 \times 100 =$ 21. $0.1 \times 0.01 =$

Division of Decimal Numbers. Round to Nearest Tenth

22. $0.25 \div 0.5 =$

23. $100 \div 1.5 =$

24. $0.667 \div 0.3 =$

25. $1.78 \div 0.04 =$

Convert into Decimal Numbers. Round to the Nearest Tenth

26. $\dfrac{4}{5} =$

27. $\dfrac{1}{2} =$

28. $\dfrac{1}{4} =$

29. $\dfrac{3}{4} =$

30. $\dfrac{16}{25} =$

31. $1\dfrac{7}{8} =$

Convert into Fractions. Simplify to their Lowest Terms

32. $0.6 =$

33. $0.57 =$

34. $1.25 =$

35. $0.01 =$

36. Arrange in size from the largest to the smallest: 0.1, 0.01, 0.001, 1.01

Convert Fractions ↔ Decimal Numbers ↔ Percents

Complete the table. Express fractions in their lowest terms.

Fraction	Decimal Number	Percent
(37)	(38)	25%
$\dfrac{5}{6}$	(39)	(40)
(41)	0.001	(42)
$1\dfrac{3}{4}$	(43)	(44)

45. Arrange in size from the smallest to the largest. 10.01, 1.901, 10.1, 1.991

Part III: Your Score: _____ /45 = _____ %

Diagnose Your Strengths and Weaknesses

Your Score/Number of Questions / Percentage

PART I	Arithmetic of whole numbers	_____	/15 =	_____ %
PART II	Arithmetic of fractions	_____	/70 =	_____ %
PART III	Arithmetic of numbers	_____	/45 =	_____ %
	TOTAL	____	/130 =	____ 100%

Did you receive 100% on each part?

No — Complete this module and do the posttest.
YES — Proceed to module 2.

Module 1: Arithmetic of Whole Numbers, Fractions, Decimal Numbers, and Percents

Module Topics

- fractions
- changing improper fractions and mixed numbers
- arithmetic of fractions
- decimal numbers
- rules for writing decimal numbers
- arithmetic of decimal numbers
- percent

Fractions
Definitions of Fractions

The word *fraction* is from the Latin fractus, meaning "broken." A fraction is a number that represents a part of a whole unit.

Example: $\dfrac{3}{4}$

The *numerator* is the top value. The *denominator* is the bottom value.

Example: $\dfrac{3}{4} \begin{array}{l} \rightarrow \text{numerator} \\ \rightarrow \text{denominator} \end{array}$

Types of Fractions

Proper fraction: the numerator is smaller in value than the denominator.

Example: $\dfrac{1}{3}$

Improper fraction: the numerator is greater in value than the denominator.

Example: $\dfrac{4}{3}$

Mixed number: a unit that contains a whole number and a fraction.

Example: $1\dfrac{1}{3}$

Equivalent fractions: Two or more fractions that have the same value but are expressed in different numbers. When the numerator and denominator are multiplied by the same number, the value of the fraction does not change. Likewise, both terms of a fraction can be divided by the same number without changing the value of the fraction. This is an important principle in the arithmetic of fractions. Many mathematical operations with fractions will require expanding and reducing.

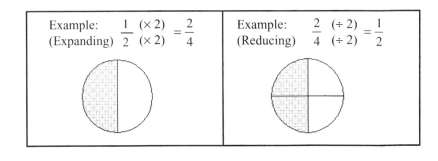

Example: (Expanding) $\dfrac{1 \ (\times 2)}{2 \ (\times 2)} = \dfrac{2}{4}$

Example: (Reducing) $\dfrac{2 \ (\div 2)}{4 \ (\div 2)} = \dfrac{1}{2}$

Lowest term: the numerator and denominator are reduced to the lowest possible value by dividing the denominator and the numerator by the same number.

NOTE: Fractions must be expressed in lowest terms.

Example: $\dfrac{1}{2}$ is in its lowest term.

$\dfrac{2}{4}$ is not expressed in its lowest term.

To simplify: 1.   Divide both the numerator and the denominator by the same number (in this example, by 2).

2.   Place the new value of the numerator over the new value of the denominator.

$$\frac{2}{4} = \frac{?}{?}$$

$$\frac{2}{4}\frac{(\div 2)}{(\div 2)} = \frac{1}{2}$$

Changing Improper Fractions and Mixed Numbers

An *improper fraction* can be changed to a *mixed number* by dividing the numerator by the denominator.

Example: $\dfrac{4}{3} = ?$

$$4 \div 3 = 1\frac{1}{3}$$

Similarly, a *mixed number* may be changed to an *improper fraction* by:

1.   Multiplying the whole number by the denominator.
2.   Adding the numerator to the product.
3.   Placing the sum over the denominator.

Example: $5\dfrac{1}{3} = ?$

$$5 \times \frac{3}{3} + 1 = \frac{16}{3}$$

Arithmetic of Fractions

Adding Fractions

To add fractions with the same denominator:

1. Add the numerators.

2. Place the sum over the denominator.

3. Simplify if necessary.

> **Example:** $\dfrac{1}{5} + \dfrac{2}{5}$
>
> $1 + 2 = 3$
>
> $\dfrac{3}{5}$

To add fractions with unlike denominators:

1. Find the common denominator. This is the smallest whole number that the denominators of the two or more fractions will divide into evenly.

2. Convert each fraction to an equivalent fraction using the common denominator.

3. Add numerators and place the sum over the common denominator.

4. Simplify the answer.

> **Example:** $\dfrac{1}{2} + \dfrac{2}{3} = ?$
>
> The common denominator is 6: both 2 and 3 divide evenly into this number.
>
> Convert: $\dfrac{1}{2} \dfrac{(\times 3)}{(\times 3)} = \dfrac{3}{6}$
>
> $\dfrac{2}{3} \dfrac{(\times 2)}{(\times 2)} = \dfrac{4}{6}$
>
> Add: $\dfrac{3}{6} + \dfrac{4}{6} = \dfrac{3+4}{6} = \dfrac{7}{6}$
>
> Simplify: $\dfrac{7}{16} = 1\dfrac{1}{6}$

Subtracting Fractions

To subtract fractions that have the same denominator:

1. Subtract the numerators.

2. Place the answer over the denominator.

3. Simplify if necessary.

> **Example:** $\dfrac{3}{4} - \dfrac{1}{4} = ?$
>
> $\dfrac{3-1}{4} = \dfrac{2}{4} = \dfrac{1}{2}$

To subtract fractions with unlike denominators:

1. Find the common denominator.

2. Convert each fraction to an equivalent fraction using the common denominator.

3. Subtract the numerators and place the difference over the common denominator.

4. Simplify if necessary.

Example: $\dfrac{5}{6} - \dfrac{3}{8} = ?$

The common denominator is 24.

Convert: $\dfrac{5}{6} = \dfrac{?}{24} \quad \dfrac{5 \ (\times 4)}{6 \ (\times 4)} = \dfrac{20}{24}$

Convert: $\dfrac{3}{8} = \dfrac{?}{24} \quad \dfrac{3 \ (\times 3)}{8 \ (\times 3)} = \dfrac{9}{24}$

Subtract: $\dfrac{20 - 9}{24} = \dfrac{11}{24}$

Simplify: $\dfrac{11}{24}$ is expressed in the lowest term.

Adding and Subtracting Mixed Numbers

To add or subtract mixed numbers:

1. Convert the mixed number to an improper fraction.

2. Follow the steps outlined for addition and subtraction of fractions.

Example: $1\dfrac{1}{3} + \dfrac{3}{4} = ?$

Convert the mixed number: $1\dfrac{1}{3}$ is $\dfrac{4}{3}$

Find the common denominator:

12 is evenly divided by both 3 and 4.

Convert: $\dfrac{4 \ (\times 4)}{3 \ (\times 4)} = \dfrac{16}{12}$

Convert: $\dfrac{3 \ (\times 3)}{4 \ (\times 3)} = \dfrac{9}{12}$

$\dfrac{16 + 9}{12} = \dfrac{25}{12}$

Convert to a mixed number:

$\dfrac{25}{12} = 2\dfrac{1}{2}$

Example: $2 - \dfrac{1}{2} = ?$

Convert the whole number to a fraction:

$2 = \dfrac{2}{1}$

Find the common denominator: 2

Convert: $\dfrac{2 \ (\times 2)}{1 \ (\times 2)} = \dfrac{4}{2}$

Subtract: $\dfrac{4 - 1}{2} = \dfrac{3}{2}$

Convert to a mixed number:

$\dfrac{3}{2} = 1\dfrac{1}{2}$

To add or subtract mixed numbers, you may also follow this example:

> **Example:** $2\frac{1}{2} + 3\frac{1}{3}$
>
> Add the whole numbers: $2 + 3 = 5$
>
> Add the fractions: $\frac{1}{2} + \frac{1}{3}$
>
> Convert to a common denominator:
>
> $$\frac{1}{2}\frac{(\times 3)}{(\times 3)} = \frac{3}{6}$$
>
> $$\frac{1}{3}\frac{(\times 2)}{(\times 2)} = \frac{2}{6}$$
>
> Add the fractions: $\frac{3+2}{6} = \frac{5}{6}$
>
> Add the whole number: $5\frac{5}{6}$

Multiplication of Fractions

<u>To multiply fractions:</u>

1. Multiply the numerators.

2. Multiply the denominators.

3. Place the product of the numerators over the product of the denominators.

4. Simplify if necessary.

> **Example:** $\frac{2}{3} \times \frac{5}{7}$
>
> $$\frac{2 \times 5}{3 \times 7} = \frac{10}{21}$$

<u>To multiply a fraction by a whole number:</u>

1. Multiply only the numerator of the fraction by the whole number.

2. Place the product over the denominator.

3. Simplify if necessary or express the whole number as a fraction and proceed as outlined.

> **Example:** $5 \times \frac{3}{7} = ?$
>
> $$\frac{5}{1} \times \frac{3}{7} = \frac{5 \times 3}{1 \times 7} = \frac{15}{7}$$
>
> Simplify: $\frac{15}{7} = 2\frac{1}{7}$

To multiply a fraction by a mixed number:

1. Change the mixed number to an improper fraction.
2. Multiply the numerators.
3. Multiply the denominators.
4. Place the product of the numerators over the product of the denominators.
5. Simplify if necessary or convert to a mixed number.

Example: $3\frac{1}{5} \times \frac{3}{4} = ?$

$$3\frac{1}{5} = \frac{16}{5}$$

$$\frac{16}{5} \times \frac{3}{4} = \frac{16 \times 3}{5 \times 4} = \frac{48}{20}$$

Simplify: $\frac{48 \; (\div 4)}{20 \; (\div 4)} = \frac{12}{5} = 2\frac{2}{5}$

Division of Fractions

To divide fractions:

1. Invert the terms of the divisor. The divisor is the number that is being divided into the dividend.

   Example: $\dfrac{1}{3} \div \dfrac{1}{2}$

   $\qquad \uparrow \qquad \uparrow$

   dividend divisor

2. Use multiplication.

Example: $\frac{1}{3} \div \frac{1}{2} = ?$

Invert the divisor: $\frac{1}{2} = \frac{2}{1}$

Multiply: $\frac{1}{3} \times \frac{2}{1} = \frac{1 \times 2}{3 \times 1} = \frac{2}{3}$

To divide a fraction by a whole number:

1. Express the whole number as a fraction.
2. Invert the divisor.
3. Use multiplication.
4. Simplify or convert to a mixed number.

Example: $\frac{5}{6} \div 2 = ?$

2 as a fraction is $\frac{2}{1}$

Invert: $\frac{2}{1}$ becomes $\frac{1}{2}$

Multiply: $\frac{5}{6} \times \frac{1}{2} = \frac{5 \times 1}{6 \times 2} = \frac{5}{12}$

To divide a fraction by a mixed number:

1. Change the mixed number to an improper fraction.
2. Invert the divisor.
3. Use multiplication.
4. Simplify if necessary.

Example: $\frac{3}{4} \div 1\frac{1}{8} = ?$

Convert to an improper fraction: $1\frac{1}{8} = \frac{9}{8}$

Invert the divisor: $\frac{9}{8} = \frac{8}{9}$

Multiply: $\frac{3}{4} \times \frac{8}{9} = \frac{3 \times 8}{4 \times 9} = \frac{24}{36}$

Simplify: $\frac{24 \; (\div 12)}{36 \; (\div 12)} = \frac{2}{3}$

Decimal Numbers

Definitions of Decimal Numbers

Decimal numbers:
- express the values that describe both whole units and portions of whole units.
- include a decimal point and values to the right and left of the decimal.
- the numbers written to the left of the decimal point are whole numbers.
- the numbers written to the right of the decimal point are decimal fractions, that is, fractions with denominators in multiples of ten.

Thus: $0.1 = \dfrac{1}{10}$ or one-tenth

$0.01 = \dfrac{1}{100}$ or one-hundredth

$0.001 = \dfrac{1}{1\,000}$ or one-thousandth

Example:
In the number 6.125 there are:

6 ones

$\dfrac{1}{10}$ or one-tenth

$\dfrac{2}{100}$ or two-hundredths

$\dfrac{5}{1\,000}$ or five-thousandths

The size of decimal numbers can be compared by examining the values in each position to the right and left of the decimal point.

Example: Which is larger, 0.5 or 0.05?

0 ones	0.5	5 tenths
0 ones	0.05	0 tenths, 5 hundredths

Therefore, 0.5 is larger than 0.05

Rules for Writing Decimal Numbers

Example: 0.25, not .25

1. Always place a zero to the left of the decimal point when there are no whole numbers.

2. Never place a zero to the right of the decimal point.

Example: 1, not 1.0
1.2, not 1.20

CRITICAL POINT

These rules are extremely important when writing drug dosages. If a drug is ordered as 0.125 mg, the zero placed before the decimal point highlights the point that might otherwise be missed. If 0.125 mg is misread as 125 mg, a fatal drug error could occur. Similarly, the zero placed after the decimal point is unnecessary. A drug order for 6 units is less likely to be misinterpreted than one written as 6.0 units. Missing the point could cause a tenfold error.

3. As with whole numbers, spaces are used to separate decimal numbers into three-digit blocks.

Example: 1.000 1
              1.078 35

Rounding Decimal Numbers

Most calibrated devices used for medication administration are accurate only to the nearest tenth or hundredth. Consequently, it is acceptable to round dosage calculations to significant digits.

To round a decimal number:

1. Locate the digit farthest to the right of the decimal point.

2. If this digit is 5 or greater, add a value of 1 to the numeral to its immediate left.

3. If this digit is less than 5, do not increase the value of the numeral to its immediate left.

4. Continue this process one digit at a time, moving right to left toward the decimal point.

Example: Round 1.125 to the nearest hundredth.

The digit in the hundredth position is 2. The digit to the right is 5. Increase the value of the numeral in the hundredth place by 1.

Answer: 1.13

Round 1.125 to the nearest tenth.

The digit in the tenth position is 1. The digit to the right is 2. Do not add a value to the tenth.

Answer: 1.1

NOTE: For most calculations, you would round to whole numbers or to tenths. In Modules 6 through 9, you will learn when to round to hundredths.

Arithmetic of Decimal Numbers

Addition and Subtraction of Decimal Numbers

Decimal points must be lined up vertically, so that tenths are under tenths, hundredths under hundredths, etc.

Addition
Example: 1.9 + 0.37 + 2.706
1.9
0.37
2.706
4.976

Subtraction
Example: 2.75 – 0.59
2.75
–0.59
2.16

Subtraction
Example: 4.2 – 3.19
4.20
–3.19
1.01

Multiplication of Decimal Numbers

The multiplication of decimal numbers follows the same rules as those for the multiplication of whole numbers, but the placement of the decimal point must be determined separately.

To multiply decimal numbers:

1. Multiply as for whole numbers.

2. Count the number of digits to the right of the decimal point in each of the numbers being multiplied.

3. Add these numbers.

4. Place the decimal point so that this number of digits is to the right of the decimal point.

Example: $2.162 \times 13.4 = ?$

2.162: 3 digits to the right of the decimal
13.4: 1 digit to the right of the decimal

The answer must have 4 digits to the right of the decimal point.

```
   2.162
×  13.4
   8648
  6486
 2162
289708
```

Place a decimal point with 4 digits to the right: 28.970 8

Division of Decimal Numbers

To divide decimal numbers:

1. Write the problem as you would for the division of whole numbers.

2. Move the decimal point to the right of the divisor, so that it becomes a whole number. This is achieved by multiplying by 10, 100, 1 000, etc.

3. Move the decimal point the same number of positions to the right in the dividend; that is, multiply both the divisor and the dividend by 10, 100, 1 000, etc.

4. Place a decimal directly above the decimal in the dividend.

5. Divide as for whole numbers.

6. Validate your answer by multiplying the answer by the divisor.

Example: $2.5\overline{)23.75}$

The divisor is 2.5; the dividend is 23.75. Multiply both the divisor and the dividend by 10:

$2.5 \times 10 = 25$
$23.75 \times 10 = 237.5$

$$
\begin{array}{r}
9.5 \\
25\overline{)237.5} \\
\underline{225} \\
12.5 \\
\underline{12.5} \\
\varnothing
\end{array}
$$

Validate: $9.5 \times 25 = 237.5$

Converting Fractions and Decimal Numbers

To convert a fraction to a decimal:

1. Divide the numerator by the denominator.

2. Round off as required.

Example: $\dfrac{1}{2} = ?$

$1 \div 2 = 0.5$

To convert a decimal number to a fraction:

1. Determine the denominator as 10, 100, 1 000, etc., by the number of digits to the right of the decimal point.

2. Express as a fraction by placing the number over the selected denominator.

3. Simplify if necessary.

Example: 0.6 has 1 digit to the right

$$= \text{tenths or } \frac{6}{10}$$

0.06 has 2 digits to the right

$$= \text{hundredths or } \frac{6}{100}$$

0.006 has 3 digits to the right

$$= \text{thousandths or } \frac{6}{1\,000}$$

Example: convert 0.06 to a fraction
The denominator is 100

$$\frac{6}{100} = \frac{3}{50}$$

To convert a mixed number to a decimal number:

1. Express the mixed number as an improper fraction.

2. Divide the numerator by the denominator.

Example: $1\frac{1}{4} = ?$

$$1\frac{1}{4} = \frac{5}{4} = 1.25$$

Percent

Percent means "parts in a hundred" $\dfrac{x}{100} = x\%$. Our most frequent encounter with percentages is with relation to exam scores. For example, if your score is 90%, you answered 90 questions out of 100 correctly. However, few exams have 100 questions — thankfully! What does percent mean when there are only 30 rather than 100 parts? The first step is to convert to an equivalent fraction. If you answered 12 questions correctly out of 30, your score would be:

Example: Express as an equivalent fraction

$$\frac{12}{30} = \frac{x}{100}$$

Solve: $30x = 1\ 200$

$$x = \frac{1\ 200}{30} = 30\overline{)1\ 200}$$
$$\phantom{x = \frac{1\ 200}{30} = 30)}\frac{40}{1\ 200}$$

Add the percent sign = 40%

Your score is 40%.

To change a decimal number to a percent:

1. Multiply the decimal by 100.

2. Add the percent sign.

Example: $0.67 = ?$
$0.67 \times 100 = 67$
67%

To change a fraction to a percent:

1. Convert the fraction to a decimal number (previously explained in this module).

2. Multiply the decimal by 100.

3. Add the percent sign.

Example: $\frac{1}{5} = ?$

$\frac{1}{5} = 0.2$

$0.2 \times 100 = 20$
20%

To change a percent to a decimal number:

1. Remove the percent sign.

2. Divide by 100.

3. Write the decimal number according to the rules.

Example: $40\% = ?$
40
$40 \div 100 = .4$
0.4

To change a percent to a fraction:

1. Place the percent number over 100.

2. Simplify if necessary.

Example: $40\% = ?$

$\frac{40}{100} = \frac{2}{5}$

POSTTEST

Instructions

Write the posttest without referring to any reference material.

Express all fractions in their lowest terms; change improper fractions to whole numbers and proper fractions.

Correct the posttest using the answer guide.

Arithmetic of Whole Numbers

1. $\begin{array}{r} 43 \\ + 68 \\ \hline \end{array}$

3. $\begin{array}{r} 37 \\ - 19 \\ \hline \end{array}$

5. $\begin{array}{r} 49 \\ \times 71 \\ \hline \end{array}$

7. $35\overline{)210}$

2. $\begin{array}{r} 140 \\ + 237 \\ \hline \end{array}$

4. $\begin{array}{r} 421 \\ - 139 \\ \hline \end{array}$

6. $\begin{array}{r} 721 \\ \times 84 \\ \hline \end{array}$

8. $210\overline{)1\,533}$

Addition of Fractions

9. $\dfrac{3}{4} + \dfrac{1}{7} =$

11. $\dfrac{3}{7} + \dfrac{1}{2} =$

13. $\dfrac{5}{12} + \dfrac{2}{10} =$

15. $\dfrac{2}{3} + \dfrac{6}{7} =$

10. $\dfrac{1}{8} + 1\dfrac{2}{5} =$

12. $14 + \dfrac{7}{12} =$

14. $\dfrac{5}{9} + \dfrac{15}{18} =$

16. $\dfrac{21}{32} + \dfrac{5}{16} =$

Subtraction of Fractions

17. $\dfrac{8}{9} - \dfrac{5}{12} =$

19. $4\dfrac{1}{5} - 3 =$

21. $\dfrac{7}{8} - \dfrac{2}{3} =$

23. $\dfrac{3}{7} - \dfrac{1}{4} =$

18. $2\dfrac{1}{2} - \dfrac{1}{6} =$

20. $21 - \dfrac{15}{16} =$

22. $\dfrac{11}{15} - \dfrac{3}{8} =$

24. $\dfrac{5}{9} - \dfrac{7}{16} =$

Multiplication of Fractions

25. $\dfrac{2}{9} \times \dfrac{3}{7} =$

27. $\dfrac{3}{4} \times 100 =$

29. $\dfrac{3}{4} \times 4 =$

31. $2 \times \dfrac{5}{8} =$

26. $1\dfrac{1}{2} \times \dfrac{2}{5} =$

28. $23 \times \dfrac{1}{3} =$

30. $1\dfrac{1}{2} \times 52 =$

32. $\dfrac{7}{16} \times \dfrac{3}{7} =$

Division of Fractions

33. $\dfrac{9}{16} \div \dfrac{3}{4} =$ 35. $\dfrac{9}{15} \div \dfrac{2}{3} =$ 37. $\dfrac{5}{9} \div \dfrac{7}{10} =$ 39. $100 \div \dfrac{3}{4} =$

34. $3\dfrac{1}{4} \div \dfrac{1}{3} =$ 36. $\dfrac{5}{6} \div 2 =$ 38. $10 \div \dfrac{3}{4} =$ 40. $2\dfrac{3}{4} \div \dfrac{1}{8} =$

Express as Improper Fractions

41. $12\dfrac{2}{3} =$

42. $3\dfrac{2}{4} =$

Change these Improper Fractions to Mixed or Whole Numbers

43. $\dfrac{21}{5} =$ 45. $\dfrac{11}{4} =$ 47. $\dfrac{203}{12} =$

44. $\dfrac{38}{9} =$ 46. $\dfrac{89}{7} =$ 48. $\dfrac{10}{3} =$

Find the Lowest Common Denominator

49. $\dfrac{7}{9}$ and $\dfrac{3}{8}$ 51. $\dfrac{13}{18}$ and $\dfrac{23}{24}$

50. $\dfrac{15}{16}$ and $\dfrac{2}{3}$ 52. $\dfrac{5}{6}$ and $\dfrac{4}{7}$

Reduce to the Lowest Terms

53. $\dfrac{16}{36} =$ 55. $\dfrac{15}{18} =$

54. $\dfrac{25}{45} =$ 56. $\dfrac{12}{4} =$

57. Which of the following is a proper fraction? Circle your choice.

$$\frac{8}{9} \qquad \frac{4}{3} \qquad 1\frac{1}{4}$$

58. Which of the following is an improper fraction? Circle you choice.

$$\frac{7}{8} \qquad \frac{21}{30} \qquad \frac{14}{11}$$

59. Which of the following is a mixed number? Circle your choice.

$$1\frac{2}{3} \qquad \frac{7}{7} \qquad \frac{5}{9}$$

Express the Following Fractions as Equivalent Fractions

60. $\dfrac{5}{7} = \dfrac{35}{?}$

62. $\dfrac{5}{9} = \dfrac{?}{108}$

64. $\dfrac{8}{11} = \dfrac{32}{?}$

61. $\dfrac{14}{35} = \dfrac{28}{?}$

63. $\dfrac{3}{20} = \dfrac{?}{200}$

Addition of Decimal Numbers. Round to the nearest hundredth.

65. $1.347 + 2.8 =$

67. $1.21 + 0.05 =$

66. $0.069 + 1.7 =$

68. $1.239 + 0.08 =$

Subtraction of Decimal Numbers. Round to the nearest tenth.

69. $3.52 - 1.19 =$

71. $18.09 - 16.9 =$

70. $8.57 - 6.68 =$

72. $3.43 - 1.009\ 7 =$

Multiplication of Decimal Numbers

73. $5.06 \times 2.1 =$

75. $2.5 \times 1.7 =$

74. $10.1 \times 0.03 =$

76. $1.01 \times 100 =$

Division of Decimal Numbers

77. $9 \div 0.05 =$

79. $0.1 \div 0.05 =$

78. $0.25 \div 2 =$

80. $12.3 \div 4.1 =$

Rounding Decimal Numbers

Round to the nearest tenth

81. 4.15

83. 1.26

82. 1.77

84. 2.33

Round to the nearest hundredth

85. 1.885

87. 10.635

86. 1.973

88. 0.359

Convert Fractions ↔ Decimal Numbers ↔ Percents

Complete the table. Express all fractions in their lowest terms.

Fraction	Decimal Number	Percent
$\frac{2}{3}$	(89)	(90)
(91)	**0.88**	(92)
(93)	(94)	**37%**
$3\frac{4}{5}$	(95)	(96)
(97)	**1.2**	(98)
(99)	(100)	**0.3%**

Your Score: _____ **/100** = _____ **%**

100%   **YES** — proceed to the next module

NO — review this module, rewrite the posttest, and obtain remedial assistance if necessary.

Module 2: Ratio and Proportion

Module Topics

- defining ratio
- expressing ratios as fractions, decimal numbers, and percents
- defining proportion
- using proportion for dosage calculation
- exercises and additional practice

There is no pretest to Module 2. If you are familiar with writing proportion statements and using ratio/proportion to solve problems, you may want to proceed to the posttest.

RATIO

Definition of Ratio

A **ratio** is a relationship that exists between two quantities. For example, a class of nursing students has 2 male and 148 female students. The ratio of males to females may be expressed as:

$$\text{a to b} \qquad \text{or} \qquad \text{a:b}$$

In this class the ratio of male to female is:

$$\text{2 to 148} \qquad \text{or} \qquad \text{2:148}$$

Stated in equivalent terms the ratio is 1 : 74

$$\left(\frac{2 \div 2}{148 \div 2} = \frac{1}{74} \right)$$

That is, for every 74 female students, there is 1 male student. (What do you think of this ratio? Your answer is probably influenced by your gender.)

In this sample, the ratio of male students to the total class would be expressed as follows:

$$\text{male : total} = 2:150$$

It is very important to be certain you are choosing the correct numbers for the ratio equation.

Example:

Out of a basket of 200 apples, 57 are red and the remaining ones are green. The ratio of red to green is 57:143

Ratios are used commonly in everyday situations. When you are jogging, swimming, or cycling, perhaps you chart your performance in kilometres per hour or metres per minute. Walking at 5 kilometres per hour will burn up almost 3 calories per minute. Five kilometres per hour and 3 calories per minute are ratios.

Ratios are frequently used in drug calculations. The dosage strength of a medication can be expressed as a ratio.

Example:

1 tablet contains 300 mg of drug.
Ratio is 300 mg per tablet, or 300:1.

Exercise 2:1

Complete the following exercise without referring to the previous test. Correct your answers by using the answer guide. (Value: 1 each)

You answered 18 questions correctly on an exam with 20 questions.

1. What is the ratio of incorrect to correct answers?
    Answer: _____

2. What is the ratio of correct to total answers?
    Answer: _____

3. The drug bottle label states, "Each tablet contains 325 units." Express the ratio of this drug in units per tablet.
    Answer: _____

4. A bottle of liquid medication states that each teaspoon contains 25 units. Express the ratio of units per teaspoon.
    Answer: _____

5. In every hour of television programming that you watch, you also "enjoy" 12 minutes of advertising. Express the following as a ratio: time of advertising, in minutes, to time of actual program, in minutes.
    Answer: _____

Your Score: _____ /5 = _____ %

Expressing Ratios as Fractions, Decimal Numbers, and Percents

A ratio may be expressed as a fraction, a decimal number, or a percent.

To convert a ratio to a fraction:

1. Place the first digit in the ratio over the second digit.

2. Simplify the fraction.

> **Example:** 2:50 as a fraction
>
> $$\frac{2}{50}$$
>
> Lowest term: $\dfrac{1}{25}$

To convert a ratio to a decimal number:

1. Express the ratio as a fraction.

2. Divide the numerator into the denominator.

3. Follow the rules for writing decimals.

> **Example:** 1:15 as a decimal
>
> Express as a fraction: $\dfrac{1}{15}$
>
> Divide: 1 divided by 15 = .066
>
> Follow rules for writing decimals: 0.066

To convert a ratio to a percent:

1. Express the ratio as a fraction.

2. Convert the fraction to a decimal number (divide numerator by denominator).

3. Multiply the decimal number by 100.

4. Add the percent sign.

> **Example:** 1:20 as a percent
>
> $$\frac{1}{20} = 0.05$$
>
> 0.05 x 100 = 5
>
> Answer: 5%

Similarly, a percent may be expressed as a ratio, since percent means "out of one hundred." To convert a percent to a ratio, place the percent over 100. Thus:

$$50\% = \frac{50}{100} = \frac{5}{10} = \frac{1}{2} = 1{:}2$$

$$0.5\% = \frac{0.5}{100} = \frac{5}{1\,000} = \frac{1}{200} = 1{:}200$$

Exercise 2.2

Complete the table without referring to the previous text. Correct your answer by using the answer guide.

Ratio	Fraction	Decimal Number	Percent
2:50	(1)	(2)	(3)
(4)	$\dfrac{1}{10}$	(5)	(6)
(7)	(8)	**0.78**	(9)
(10)	(11)	(12)	**33.3**
(13)	$\dfrac{50}{1}$	(14)	(15)

Your Score: _____ **/15** = _____ **%**

PROPORTION

Definition of Proportion

Proportion: expression of two equal or equivalent ratios. The two ratios are separated by an equal sign. For example, 2:3 = 4:6. In a true proportion, the product of the mean equals the product of the extremes: thus,

$$\underset{\text{extremes}}{\overset{\text{means}}{2:3 = 4:6}}$$

$$2 \times 6 = 3 \times 4$$
$$12 = 12$$

NOTE: the *m*eans are the values in the *m*iddle, the *e*xtremes are the values on the *e*nds.

9:3 = 6:2	8:4 = 4:2
because	because
$9 \times 2 = 3 \times 6$	$8 \times 2 = 4 \times 4$
$18 = 18$	$16 = 16$

Using Proportion for Dosage Calculation

A proportion equation can be used to solve for an unknown quantity. The proportion equation is the simplest and most accurate approach to calculating drug dosages. In these situations, you have a known ratio; for example, the drug label states 325 mg per tablet or a ratio of 325:1. Another label states 100 mg in 2 mL or 100 mg:2 mL. The dosage that you wish to give is the unknown ratio. You know what strength to give, but you must determine the volume to give (the number of tablets or millilitres, for example.)

To solve for an unknown value (x) using proportion:

1. Write the known ratio first.

2. Write the unknown ratio.

3. Set up the proportion.

4. Multiply the means and the extremes; place the unknown value on the left.

5. Solve for the unknown. Recall that you must divide both sides of an equation by the same number.

6. Validate your answer. Prove the answer.

Example: 200:4 = 500:x

$200 \times x = 4 \times 50$
$200x = 200$
$x = 1$

Validation: 200:4 = 50:1

$200 \times 1 = 4 \times 50$
$200 = 200$

Dosage calculations using proportion equations are illustrated in Modules 5 through 9. Proceed to exercise 2.3 to practice setting up proportions.

Proportion: Alternative Solution

You may be more familiar with writing a proportion as two fractions and using "cross multiplication."

To solve for an unknown value (x) using fractions as proportion:

1. Write the known ratio as a fraction.

2. Write the unknown ratio as a fraction using x for the unknown value.

3. Determine the cross product: multiply the numerator of each by the denominator of the other fraction.

4. Solve for x. Divide both sides of the equation by the same value.

5. Validate your answer by substituting the value for x into the original equation.

Example: 5:10 = 7:x

$$\frac{5}{10} = \frac{7}{x} \qquad \frac{5}{10} \diagup\!\!\!\times \frac{7}{x}$$

$5x = 70$

$$\frac{5x}{5} = \frac{70}{5}$$

$x = 14$

Validate:
5:10 = 7:14

$$\frac{5}{10} = \frac{7}{14}$$

$70 = 70$

Exercise 2.3

Complete the following exercise without referring to the previous text. Correct using the answer guide. Express answers in whole or decimal numbers. Round to nearest hundredth. (Questions 1-15, Value: 1 each)

Solve for x:

1. $2:3 = x:12$

2. $1:5 = x:125$

3. $5:7 = 15:x$

4. $25:1 = 50:x$

5. $10:1 = 15:x$

6. $75:6 = 50:x$

7. $35:x = 100:1$

8. $0.25:1 = 0.125x$

9. $250:1\,000 = x:1$

10. $10:1\,000 = x:100$

11. $1:8 = 1/2:x$

12. $18:x = 5:300$

13. $0.5:2 = x:4$

14. $1/4:x = 6:12$

15. $x:6 = 1/100:1/10$

For each of the following problems, show your work and validate the answer (show the proof). (Value: 2 each, 1 for right answer, 1 for validation)

16. To make 6 cups of coffee, you use 4 scoops of coffee and water. How many scoops do you need to make 24 cups?
     Answer: _____

17. The pancake recipe requires 1 cup of milk and 1 1/2 cups of mix. You have 6 cups of mix. How much milk should you add?
     Answer: _____

18. You are making party bags for the birthday and want to put in 1 package of gum with 3 packages of mints. How many packages of gum do you need for 45 packages of mints?
     Answer: _____

19. At the last hotdog day, 22 children ate 33 hotdogs. How many hotdogs will you prepare for a class of 28 children?
     Answer: _____

20. The fruit drink recipe calls for 1 cup of lime juice to 3 cups of apple juice. How much lime juice will you add to 24 cups of apple juice?
     Answer: _____

Your Score: _____ **/25** = _____ %

Exercise 2.4

Solve for x. (Value: 1 each)

Express answers as whole or decimal numbers.

1. $3 : x = 1 : 15$

4. $\dfrac{25}{1} = \dfrac{100}{x}$

2. $9 : x = 3 : 4$

5. $\dfrac{8}{x} = \dfrac{12}{6}$

3. $\dfrac{x}{100} = \dfrac{5}{20}$

6. $\dfrac{1}{50} = \dfrac{x}{150}$

Express the following ratios as fractions, decimal numbers, and percents. Reduce fractions to lowest term. (Value: 1 each)

Ratio	Fraction	Decimal Number	Percent
1:100	(7)	(8)	(9)
1 : 5	(10)	(11)	(12)
4:1 000	(13)	(14)	(15)

Solve for x. (Value: 1 each)

16. $\dfrac{0.25}{1} = \dfrac{0.125}{x}$

18. $\dfrac{1\,000}{1.5} = \dfrac{x}{3}$

17. $\dfrac{2.2}{1} = \dfrac{x}{75}$

19. $60 : 5 = 150 : x$

20. You buy 7 oranges and 5 apples. What is the ratio of oranges to apples?

     Answer: _____

21. There are 40 patients and 8 staff members. What is the ratio of patients to staff? Express as a ratio in lowest terms. (Value: 2)

     Answer: _____

22. Your score is 85% on a math exam. What is the ratio of correct to incorrect answers? Express as a ratio in lowest terms. (Value: 2)

    Answer: _____

23. Your coffeemaker instructions state that 6 scoops of coffee make 8 cups of coffee. How many scoops are needed to make 2 cups? (Value: 2)

    Answer: _____

24. Define the term *ratio*. (Value: 2)

25. Define the term *proportion*. (Value: 2)

For each problem, write the proportion equation and solve for x. (Value: 2 each)

26. There are 2 baskets of fruit with equal ratios of oranges and apples. Basket 1 has 3 oranges and 5 apples. Basket 2 has 9 oranges. How many apples are there in Basket 2?

27. Two classes of children are going on a field trip, and you want the same ratio of children from grades 2 and 3 in each bus. The first bus has 8 grade 2 students and 12 grade 3 students. The second bus has 10 grade 2 students. How many grade 3 students should there be in the second bus?

28. A basketball player has a scoring average of 18 out of 25 shots. How many baskets will she likely score if she takes 50 shots?

29. The recipe calls for 1 cup of milk and 2 cups of flour. How much milk should be used for 3 cups of flour?

30. A necklace has 5 blue beads to 12 red beads. How many blue beads should there be for 48 red beads?

Your Score: _____ /40 = _____ %

POSTTEST

Instructions

Write the posttest without referring to any reference materials.

Correct the posttest using the answer guide.

Solve for x.

1. 3:7 = x:21   x =

2. $\dfrac{x}{10} = \dfrac{4}{5}$ x =

3. 1:10 = x :100   x =

4. Of 62 students in psychology, 23 are male. What is the ratio of male students to female students?
    Answer: _____

5. A hockey player scores 3 goals in 17 shots. What is the ratio of goals to shots?
    Answer: _____

6. There are 28 patients on a particular ward. The ratio of staff to patients is 1 to 4. How many staff members are on this ward?
    Answer: _____

7. Define the term *ratio*.

8. Define the term *proportion*.

9. Express the following statement as a ratio.
    Each teaspoon contains ten units of Drug A.
    Answer: _____

10. Is the following relationship a proportion?
    6:32 = 24:100   Yes or No

11. Express 0.9% as a ratio.
    Answer: _____

Express the following ratios as fractions, decimal numbers, and percents. Express fractions in lowest terms and round decimal numbers to the nearest tenth.

Ratio	Fraction	Decimal Number	Percent
1:1	(12)	(13)	(14)
(15)	$\dfrac{2}{3}$	(16)	(17)
(18)	(19)	0.001	(20)

Express these ratios as fractions. Simplify if necessary.

21. 12:1 000

22. 16:500

23. 7:56

24. 26:65

Write the true proportion for each of the following statements. Show the proportion statement, the work to achieve the solution, and validation of the answer.

There are 12 red beads, and the pendant has 1 red bead for every 8 green beads. How many green beads are on the pendant?

25. Proportion statement.

26. Solution.

27. Validation.

The salt solution has 1.5 tablespoons of salt in 3 cups of water. How much salt is needed for 8 cups?

28. Proportion statement.

29. Solution.

30. Validation.

Your Score: _____ /30 = _____ %

100% YES — proceed to the next module

NO — review this module, rewrite posttest, and obtain remedial assistance if necessary.

Note: If you had any errors on the posttest, analyze your areas of weakness before reviewing.

Module 3: Systems of Measurement

Module Topics

- systems of measurement
    - household
    - apothecary
    - SI
- rules for writing SI
- converting written SI
- common conversions between systems
- temperature conversions
- exercises

Systems of Measurement

In the past, pharmacology has relied on several systems of measurement that have made dosage calculations quite confusing.

This confusion has contributed to medication errors. Today the movement is towards standardization. All drugs should be ordered and dispensed in SI units. Drug orders should be written in units called *grams*, *milligrams*, and *millilitres*. Nurses should not have to do conversions from one system of measurement to another, except for a few instances involving liquid medications, such as laxatives or antacids, or for instructions to the patient and family regarding uses of over-the-counter (OTC) drugs.

CRITICAL POINT

If you are unfamiliar with any drug order written in nonstandardized units, consult with the prescribing physician or a pharmacist.

Three major systems of measurement have been used in pharmacology. They are the household system, the apothecary system and the metric system.

Household System

This system uses measures such as *drops*, *teaspoons*, and *tablespoons*. These measurements are most frequently used for prescription medications taken in the home and with such drugs as eye medications in the hospital.

Apothecary System

This is a very old system whose basic units include *minims, ounces,* and *grains.* These measures have almost become obsolete except for some drug orders for laxatives, antacids, and cough syrups that may be written in ounces.* It's useful for you to be familiar with some of the units of these systems, since patients and families might be accustomed to these measures.† However, the official system of measurement in Canada is the SI system, and, therefore, emphasis is placed on this system in the module.

SI System

The SI system or Le Systèm International D'Unités, is essentially an expanded version of the metric system. It is a decimal system based on the number 10.

There are seven base units or building blocks in this system. The *base units* you will encounter most often in relation to medications are outlined in Table 3-1.

Table 3-1: Common Base Units

Name	Unit	Symbol
metre	unit of length	m
kilogram	unit of mass	kg
mole	unit of substance	mol

You are probably familiar with *metre* and *kilogram.* You've no doubt bought a metre of fabric or driven 100 kilometres. A metre is approximately the distance between the bottom of a door and its doorknob. Possibly you have bought a kilogram of meat. A kilogram is approximately equal in weight to a 1-litre carton of milk.

A *mole* is probably familiar to you. It isn't a measurement of weight. A mole is an "amount of substance" defined as the number of atoms in exactly 12g of the carbon-12 isotope. The number of atoms in a mole of a substance is 6.02×10^{23}. If your curiosity is aroused by this definition, you might appreciate a further explanation. An anonymous and creative author described 1 mole of peas as follows:

10^{23} average-size peas would cover 250 planets the size of Earth with a blanket of peas 1 metre deep!

Obviously, 1 mole of peas occupies a much larger volume than 1 mole of the electrolyte potassium chloride.

---

* Also some aspirin products, which are still labeled in grains.
† *Pounds* and *inches* are also part of this system.

Body fluid chemistry reports are expressed in molar units. This will become more significant to you when you read drug plasma levels reported in moles.

Examples:

insulin: 30–170 pmol/L
               (picomoles per litre)

digoxin: < 2.6 nmol/L
               (nanomoles per litre)

lithium: 0.6–1.2 nmol/L
               (millimoles per litre)

NOTE: laboratory values can vary slightly. Check the normal values written on the lab reports in your particular clinical setting.

In addition to these base units, one other measurement is not an official SI unit but is of interest to health professionals. This is the unit of volume called the *litre*. For example, intravenous fluids are packaged in one litre (1 000 millilitre) containers.

Because the metre, kilogram, mole and litre are relatively large units, the SI system uses prefixes to denote multiples and subunits. There are 16 prefixes, but only those used most frequently in relation to drug therapy are written in Table 3-2.

These numerical values are very important when converting base units and subunits of the SI system. You will do this frequently when administering medications and intravenous fluids to your patients. Mastering this module is an important step toward competence in calculating dosages.

Table 3-2: SI Subunits

Prefix	Symbol	Numerical Value
kilo	k	1 000
hecto	h	100
deci	d	0.1
centi	c	0.01
milli	m	0.001
micro	μ or mc	0.000 001
nano	n	0.000 000 001
pico	p	0.000 000 000 001

NOTE: the official symbol for *micro* is μ; however some references use mc. Both abbreviations are acceptable.

Exercise 3.1

Review Table 3-2. Complete the following exercise without referring to the previous text. Correct using the answer guide. (Value: 1 each unless otherwise indicated)

Give the SI symbol for each of the following prefixes:

1. kilo   K
2. deci   d
3. centi   c
4. milli   m
5. micro   µ

Write out the numerical value for each of the following prefixes:

6. kilo   1000
7. nano
8. pico
9. milli   0.001
10. micro   0.000 001
11. centi   0.01
12. hecto   100
13. Name the 8 subunits, as outlined in Table 3-2, from largest to smallest. (Value: 8)

Your Score: _____ /20 = _____ %

Rules for Writing SI Symbols

1. Symbols of units are written in lower case initials, except when they are named after a person.

    Example:
    degree Celsius = °C
    metre = m

2. Symbols are not pluralized. They are written without a period, except when the symbol occurs at the end of a sentence.

    Example:
    He weighs 10 kg.
    Ten kg is correct.

3. Decimals should be used instead of fractions.

> **Example:**
>
> $\frac{1}{2}$ is 0.5

4. Always place a zero before the decimal point when there is no whole number.

> **Example:**
> 0.5 not .5

5. Just when you think you have this mastered, it turns out there is an exception to the rules. To avoid confusion with the number 1, write the word *litre* in full or use capital *L*. The capital *L* is also used with prefixes.

> **Example:**
> litre = L
> millilitre = mL

6. Writing numbers with more than three digits — that is, in the thousands — is slightly different from the traditional method. No comma is used. Instead a space is left, as shown in the example.

> **Example:**
> 1 000.039 78
> 23 000
> 217 860

Note: The Metric Commission of Canada states that spaces are used to separate long numbers into three-digit blocks. With four-digit numbers, the space is optional.

7. Because old habits die slowly, there is one other point you should know. Although cc, *cubic centimetre*, isn't a standard SI unit, it's frequently used by health professionals — especially those of us who are BSI — before SI! The cc should be replaced by mL (for millilitre); 1cc is approximately equal to 1 mL.

Exercise 3.2

Complete the following exercise without referring to the previous text. Correct using the answer guide. (Value: 1 each)

Indicate which of the following correctly adhere to the rules for writing SI symbols. Circle your choice.

1. metre = m or M

2. 10 kilograms = 10 kg or 10 kgs

3. $\frac{1}{2}$ millilitre = $\frac{1}{2}$ mL or 0.5 mL

4. litre = L or l

5. one thousand millilitres = 1 000 mL or 1.000 mL

6. One-half litre = .5 L or 0.5 L or 0.5 l

7. One thousand and fifty milligrams = 1 050 mgms or 1 050 mg

8. millilitre = mL or ml

9. Write fifty-one thousand, five hundred seventeen according to the SI rules.

10. True or false? 1 cc is approximately equal to 1 mL.

Your Score: _____ /10 = _____ %

Converting SI Subunits to Base Units

The most common subunits encountered in drug therapy are *milli* and *micro*. In addition, you will frequently encounter *centi* in measurements of height or length. Table 3-3 illustrates some relationships involving units of the SI system.

Table 3-3: Units and Values

Unit	Value
gram (g) to milligram (mg)	1 g = 1 000 mg
gram (g) to microgram (μg or mcg)	1 g = 1 000 000 μg (or mcg)
milligram (mg) to microgram (mg or mcg)	1 mg = 1 000 μg (or mcg)
litre (L) to millilitre (mL)	1 L = 1 000 mL
metre (m) to centimetre (cm)	1 m = 100 cm
metre (m) to millimetre (mm)	1 m = 1 000 mm

CRITICAL POINT

When handwriting abbreviations, write mcg to avoid confusion with mg.

Conversion of subunits to base units and vice versa is a very simple exercise, involving multiplication or division by 10, 100, or 1 000. The trick of course, is to remember whether to multiply or divide! The simplest approach is to use a proportion equation to solve. For example, how are grams converted to milligrams?

Method A — Proportion

Example: 10 g = x mg
Known ratio is 1 g = 1 000 mg
Unknown ratio is 10 g = x mg
  1 g:1 000 mg = 10 g:x mg
    1x = 1 000 × 10
    x = 10 000
    10 g = 10 000 mg
Validation:
1 g: 1 000 mg = 10 g:10 000 mg
1 × 10 000 = 1 000 × 10
10 000 = 10 000

Method B — Cross Product

Example: 10g = x mg

Known ratio is $\dfrac{1\ g}{1\ 000\ mg}$

Unknown ratio is $\dfrac{10\ g}{x\ mg}$

$\dfrac{1\ g}{1\ 000\ mg} = \dfrac{10\ g}{x\ mg}$

Use cross multiplication
1x = 10 × 1 000
x = 10 000 mg

Remember to write the proportion with the known ratio on the left, the unknown ratio on the right. Be sure that each side of the equation is set up in the same way. In the previous example, the known ratio is stated as g:mg, so the unknown ratio must also be stated as g:mg. Examine the following problem and determine the various ways that the proportion could be stated.

How many milligrams are there in 0.2 g?

There are at least three ways to state a proportion equation to solve this question. In each proportion, the relationship is the same for both sides of the equation.

a. 1 g:1 000 mg = 0.2 g:x mg

b. 1 g:0.2 g = 1 000 mg:x mg

c. 1 000 mg:1 g = x mg:0.2 g

Solutions for each equation show that the proportion equations all yield the same answer.

Method A — Proportion

a. 1 g:1 000 mg = 0.2 g:x mg
   1 x = 1 000 × 0.2
   x = 200
Answer is 200 mg
Validation: 1 g: 1 000 mg = 0.2 g:200 mg
   1 × 200 = 1 000 × 0.2
   200 = 200

b. 1 g:0.2 g = 1 000 mg:x mg
   1 x = 0.2 × 1 000
   x = 200
Answer is 200 mg
Validation: 1 g:0.2 g = 1 000 mg:200 mg
   1 × 200 = 0.2 × 1 000
   200 = 200

c. 1 000 mg:1 g = x mg:0.2 g
   1 x = 1 000 × 0.2
   x = 200
Answer is 200 mg
Validation: 1 000 mg:1 g = 200 mg:0.2 g
   1 000 × 0.2 = 1 × 200
   200 = 200

Method B — Cross Product

a. $\dfrac{1\ g}{1\ 000\ mg} = \dfrac{0.2\ g}{x\ mg}$
x = 1 000 × 0.2
x = 200
Validation
$\dfrac{1\ g}{1\ 000\ mg} = \dfrac{0.2\ g}{200}$
200 = 200

b. $\dfrac{1\ g}{0.2\ g} = \dfrac{1\ 000\ mg}{x\ mg}$
x = 0.2 × 1 000
x = 200
Validation
$\dfrac{1\ g}{0.2\ g} = \dfrac{1\ 000\ mg}{200\ mg}$
200 = 200

c. $\dfrac{1\ 000\ mg}{1\ g} = \dfrac{x\ mg}{0.2\ g}$
x = 1 000 × 0.2
x = 200
Validation
$\dfrac{1\ 000\ mg}{1\ g} = \dfrac{200\ mg}{0.2\ g}$
200 = 200

Exercise 3.3

Complete the following exercise without referring to the previous text. Correct using the answer guide. (Value: 1 each)

1. 1 L = _1000_ mL
2. 1 kg = _1000_ g
3. 1 m = _100_ cm
4. 1 cc = _1_ mL
5. 1 g = _1,000,000_ µg

6. 250 mL = _.25_ L
7. 0.5 g = _.50_ L
8. 2 m = _200_ cm
9. 1 mg = _1,000_ µg
10. 1 000 µg = _.1_ g

11. 300 mg = ___.3___ g ✓

12. 800 g = ___.8___ kg ✓

13. 150 cm = ___1.5___ m ✓

14. 0.75 g = ___750___ mg ✓

Your Score: ___12___ /14 = ___65___ %

Common Conversions

Because of the common usage of inches, pounds, and fluid ounces by the public and professionals, it is practical to know the following conversions from the SI system to the household and apothecary systems. Table 3-4 lists these common conversions.

Table 3-4: Common Conversions

Unit	SI	Household/Apothecaries
weight	**kg**	**pounds**
	1 kg =	2.2 pounds (lbs)
height	**cm**	**inches**
	2.54 cm =	1 inch (in)
volume	**mL**	**teaspoon**
	5 mL =	1 teaspoon (tsp)
	mL	**tablespoon**
	15 mL =	1 tablespoon (tbsp)
	mL	**fluid ounces**
	30 mL =	1 fluid ounce
	500 mL =	1 pint
	1 000 mL =	1 quart

Example: how do you convert 2 kg to it equivalent in lbs?
1 kg:2.2 lbs = 2 kg: x lbs
x = 2.2 × 2
x = 4.4
Answer is 4.4 lbs.

Example:
88 lbs = x kg
1 kg:2.2 lbs = x kg:88 lbs
2.2 x = 88
2.2 x (÷ 2.2) = 88 (÷ 2.2)
x = 40
Answer is 40 kg.

Example: 3 oz = x mL
1 oz: 30 mL = 3 oz: xmL
x = 30 × 3
x = 90
Answer is 90 mL.

Exercise 3.4

Review Table 3.4 and master the conversions before completing the following exercise. Answer the questions without referring to Table 3.4. Correct using the answer guide.

You are admitting Mr. Jones, who cannot be weighed. He tells you that his weight is 175 lb.

1. Convert Mr. Jones' weight to kgs.

2. Round to the nearest tenth.

3. Round to the nearest kg.

Tim's height is 140 cm.

4. Express Tim's height in inches.

5. Express Tim's height in feet and inches.

6. The label states, "For ages 2 to 3, give 1 tsp." Convert this measurement to mL.

7. The order is: Magnolax 1 oz. Convert to mL.

8. Jane's height is 5 feet, 3 inches; express her height in cm.

9. The label reads, "10 mL for ages 10-12." Convert this measurement to teaspoons.

10. The bottle contains 1 and 1/2 pints. Convert this to mL.

Convert. Round to nearest tenth.

11. 27 kg =   _____ lb

12. 3 tsp =   _____ mL

13. 30 inches =   _____ cm

14. 4.3 kg =   _____ lb

15. 5 feet, 6 inches = ___ cm

16. 2 fluid oz. =   _____ mL

17. 149 lbs. =   _____ kg

18. 1 quart =   _____ mL

19. 154 cm =   _____ inches

20. 240 mL =   _____ fluid oz

Your Score: _____ /20 = _____ %

Temperature Conversions

Two facts should be kept in mind when converting temperatures between Fahrenheit and Celsius. First, the freezing point of water is **0°C and 32°F.** Second, each degree Celsius is almost 2° Fahrenheit, in fact, 1°C = 1.8°F exactly. You should always take these two facts into consideration when converting.

To convert from °C to °F:
1.   Multiply by 1.8.
2.   Add 32.

Example: 40°C = ___°F
40 × 1.8 = 72
72 + 32 = 104
40°C = 104°F

Example: 36.4°C = ___°F:
36.4 × 1.18 = 65.52
65.52 + 32 = 97.5
36.4°C = 97.5°F (rounded to tenth)

Example: –5°C = ___°F
–5 × 1.8 = –9
–9 + 32 = 23
–5°C = 23°F

To convert from °F to °C:
1.   Subtract 32.
2.   Divide by 1.8.

Example: 105.3°F = ___°C
106.3 – 32 = 73.3
73.3 ÷ 1.8 = 41.7
105.3°F = 41.7°C

Example: 98.6°F = ___°C
98.6 – 32 = 66.6
66.6 ÷ 1.8 = 37
98.6°F = 37°C

Example: 19°F = ___°C
19 – 32 = –13
–13 ÷ 1.8 = –7
19°F = –7°C

NOTE: one conversion is the reverse operation in the reverse order from the other!

Exercise 3.5

Convert each of the following temperatures. Round off to the nearest tenth.

1. 39.8°C = _____ °F   2. 104.1°F = _____ °C   3. 36°C = _____ °F
4. 100.4°F = _____ °C   5. 52°F = _____ °C   6. 24°C = _____ °F
7. -8°F = _____ °C   8. -12°C = _____ °F   9. 12°F = _____ °C

Your Score: _____ /9 = _____ %

Exercise 3.6

Correct using the answer guide. (Value: 1 each)

Convert each of the following measurements:

1. 10 g = _____ mg
2. 50 mg = _____ g
3. 0.25 g = _____ mg
4. 1.25 mg = _____ micrograms (mcg)
5. 1 L = _____ mL
6. 2 kg = _____ g
7. 350 mg = _____ g
8. 1.5 m = _____ cm
9. 0.7 g = _____ mcg

Convert the following household measurements to SI units. Round to nearest whole number.

10. 3.4 fl oz = _____ mL
11. 2 tsp = _____ mL
12. 35 kg = _____ lb
13. 143 lb = _____ kg
14. 26 in = _____ cm
15. 42 cm = _____ in
16. 32 oz = _____ mL
17. 72 oz = _____ mL

18. 135 lbs = _____ kg

19. 15 mL = _____ tsp

20. 78 cm = _____ in

Your Score: _____ **/20** = _____ **%**

Exercise 3.7

In the metric system, name the base units of:

	name	abbreviation
1. length		
2. weight (mass)		
3. substance		

Give the numerical value for each prefix:

4. deci _____

5. centi _____

6. milli _____

7. nano _____

8. micro _____

9. kilo _____

Do the following conversions of SI units:

10. 1 g = _____ mg   11. 1 L = _____ mL

12. 10 mg = _____ g   13. 1 kg = _____ g

14. 1 mg = _____ g   15. 250 mL = _____ L

16. 40 g = _____ kg   17. 200 mg = _____ g

18. 0.3 g = _____ mg   19. 1 m = _____ cm

20. 250 cm = _____ m   21. 0.6 g = _____ mg

Convert the following household measurements to SI units:

22. 2 fl oz. = _____ mL   23. 1 tsp = _____ mL

24. 3 kg = _____ lb   25. 6 ft = _____ cm

Your Score: _____ /25 = _____ %

POSTTEST

Instructions

Write the posttest without referring to any reference materials.

Correct the posttest using the answer guide.

1. 2L = _____ mL

2. 250 mg = _____ g

3. 2 000 mg = _____ g

4. 6 g = _____ mg

5. 7 kg = _____ g

6. 5 000 mL = _____ L

7. 1.25 mg = _____ g

8. 0.003 g = _____ mg

9. 2.5 g = _____ mg

10. 0.5 L = _____ mL

11. 1 456 g = _____ kg

12. 0.5 mg = _____ g

13. 1 mg = _____ µg

14. 1.7 m = _____ cm

15. 179 cm = _____ m

16. 0.5 g = _____ µg

17. 250 mL = _____ L

18. 1.34 g = _____ mg

19. 10 g = _____ ug

20. 79 kg = _____ mg

Give the numerical value for each prefix:

21. centi

22. milli

23. micro

24. kilo

25. deci

Common conversions:

26. 2 tsp. = _____ mL

27. 6 fluid oz =_____ mL

28. 8 lbs. = _____ kg

29. 10 kg = _____ lbs

30. 80 cm = _____ in

31. 68°F = _____ °C

32. 6 feet, 1 inch = _____ cm

33. 38.6°C = _____ °F

34. 25 kg = _____ lbs

35. 480 mL = _____ quarts

36. 208 lbs = _____ kg

37. 75°F =   _____ °C

38. 3 tbsp. =   _____ mL

39. 1.5 quarts = _____ mL

40. 37°C =   _____ °F

Your Score: _____ /40   =   _____ %

100%   **YES** — proceed to the next module

NO — review this module, rewrite the posttest, and obtain remedial assistance if necessary.

Module 4: Medication Orders and Dosage Forms

Module Topics

- reading medication orders
- commonly-used abbreviations
- packaging of medications and dosage forms
- types of solutions
- reading medication labels

Reading Medication Orders

In most clinical settings, medications are prescribed by a physician, dispensed by a pharmacist, and administered by a nurse. All medication orders should include the patient's name, drug, dose, route, frequency or time of administration, date, and physician's signature.

NOTE: dose and dosage both refer to the exact amount of medicine to be given or taken at a specified time.

CRITICAL POINT

The major cause of medication errors is misreading or misinterpreting drug orders. Calculating dosages as well as reading and interpreting orders requires 100% accuracy.

Commonly Used Abbreviations

The first step in achieving this accuracy is correct interpretation of the medication order. Handwriting jokes aside, even a legible order is usually written in shorthand. It's important to learn this "new language." Abbreviations vary considerably among institutions and prescribers. Some are easily misinterpreted and can lead to error. For example, qd, and od have all been used to mean "daily" or "once a day." However, od also means "right eye." The abbreviation, qd, can also be confused with qid, which would result in a very serious error. For example, digoxin (Lanoxin) would be given four times a day instead of only once. The letter "u" for units can be easily misread as an "o." For example, serious drug errors have occurred because 6 u of insulin was read as 60. The abbreviations listed in Box 4 - 1 have become widely accepted. Some have been used in the calculation problems in this workbook. You are urged to verify acceptable abbreviations used in the practice setting.

Box 4-1 Commonly Used Abbreviations

ac	before meals (1/2 hour before meals)
ad lib	as desired; freely
amp.	ampoule
bid	twice daily
c̄	with
cap.	capsule
dil.	dilute
elix.	elixir
ext.	extract
gtt	drop
h, hr	hour
hs	at bedtime
IM or im	intramuscular
inh.	inhaler
IV or iv	intravenous
mcg	microgram
mEq	milliequivalent
mg	milligram
pc	after meals (1/2 hour after meals)
PO or po	by mouth
PR	per rectum
prn	as necessary (according to necessity)
qh	every hour
q4h	every 4 hours
qid	4 times a day
qs	as much as required
SC or sc	subcutaneous
SL	sublingual
sol	solution
SR	slow or sustained release
stat.	immediately
supp.	suppository
susp.	suspension
tab.	tablet
tid	3 times a day
U or iu	unit, international unit
ung.	ointment

NOTE:

Sometimes these abbreviations are written with periods; for example, b.i.d., p.o.

Unit: a drug measure based on a specific effect; for example, a unit of insulin is a standardized amount that lowers blood sugar.

Milliequivalent: measurement of combining power rather than weight.

Exercise 4.1

Complete the following exercise without referring to the previous text. Correct using the answer guide.

Interpret the following medication orders. Write out each of the underlined abbreviations in full. (Value: 3 each)

1. Meperidine (Demerol) 50–75 mg <u>IM q3–4h prn</u>
2. Acetaminophen (Tylenol) 650 mg <u>PO q4h</u>
3. Codeine sulfate 60 mg <u>PO stat and q4h</u>
4. Penicillin 500 000 units <u>IV qid</u>
5. Phenobarbital <u>elix. 100 mg hs</u>
6. List the seven parts of a medication order. (Value: 7)

Write in full the meaning for each of the abbreviations. (Value: 1 each)

7. ad lib _____
8. gtt _____
9. SL _____
10. supp _____
11. pc _____
12. tab _____
13. bid _____
14. hs _____
15. ung _____

16. mg _____
17. mcg _____
18. sc _____
19. ext. _____
20. ac _____
21. IM _____
22. qs _____
23. c̄ _____
24. stat _____

Your Score: _____ /40 = _____ %

Packaging of Medications and Dosage Forms

Medications are prepared and packaged in a variety of forms. Oral doses are provided in compressed tablets, capsules, and liquids. Some tablets are scored and can be easily broken in half. Injectables are packaged in both single-dose and multiple-dose containers. Figures 4-1 and 4-2 illustrate various packaging of drugs.

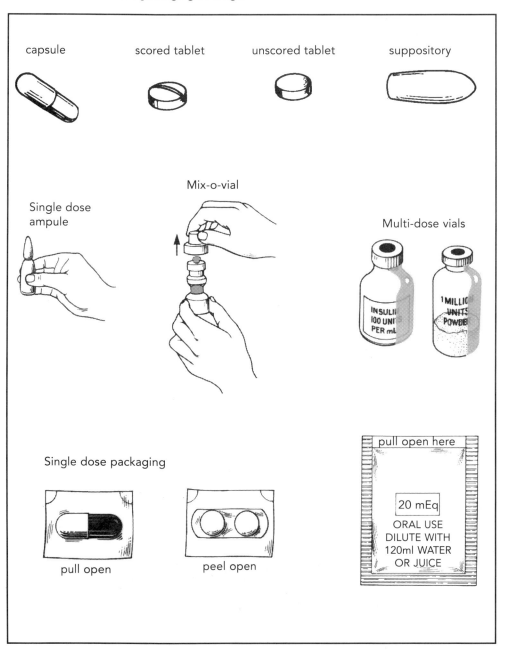

Figure 4-1 Packaging and dosage forms

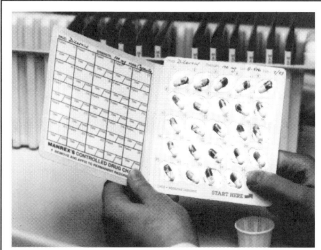

Controlled Drug System

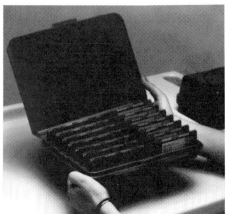

Controlled Dosage System

The Perso Care System

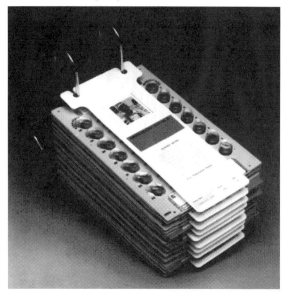

Figure 4-2 Unit-dose packaging systems (Courtesy Manrex Limited, Winnipeg, Manitoba)

CRITICAL POINT

An important point should be made about the single-dose ampule. The ampule may state that 1 mg per mL is contained and premixed for a single dose. However, the ampule contains slightly more than 1 mL, to allow for some loss of solution within the needle and syringe. Therefore, always carefully calculate and measure the correct dose and do not draw up the entire contents of an ampule. A similar point can be made regarding vials and bags of intravenous fluids. All packages of liquid medication contain extra fluid.

Injectables are prepared as liquids ready for injection or in powdered form requiring reconstitution with a diluent. The procedure for reconstitution and calculation of these products is described in Module 6.

Many drugs are prepared in liquid form. The following discussion briefly reviews terminology associated with solutions.

Types of Solutions

Definitions

A **solution** is a homogeneous mixture that contains one or more dissolved substances in a liquid. For example, when you add sugar to your tea you are creating a solution.

A **solvent** is the liquid in which another substance is dissolved. In the above example, the tea is the solvent.

A **solute** is the substance dissolved in the solvent. In our example, sugar is a solute.

Some drugs are available in solution; the drug is the solute, and water is usually the solvent. In other instances, solvents used include normal saline, alcohol, or other liquids.

When drugs are prepared in solution, they are described by the **strength** or **concentration** of the solution. The strength or concentration of a solution is determined by the amount of solute dissolved in a given amount of solvent. For example, did you put 1 tsp or 2 tsp of sugar in your cup of tea?

An example of strength of solutions is demonstrated by the preparation of heparin, which is done in varying strengths such as 1 000 units per mL and 10 000 units per mL. The latter preparation is 10 times greater in concentration than the former.

There are many types of solutions and in most instances involving drugs, they are premixed. The two types of solutions that are relevant in medication therapy are illustrated in Figure 4-3.

Weight per volume solution: the solute is weighed, but the solvent is expressed in volume: g to mL. This is the most common type of medication solution. Most intravenous solutions are expressed as a weight per volume type of solution: a given weight of dextrose, in g, is dissolved in a certain volume of water, in mL.

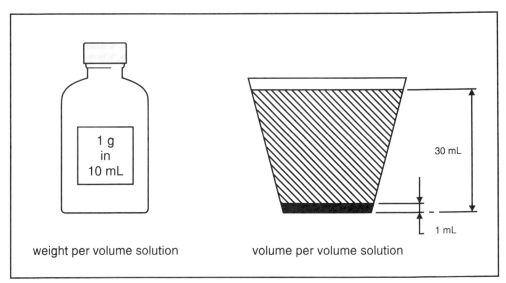

Figure 4-3 Types of solutions

Volume per volume solution: both the solute and the solvent are measured in the same units of volume. For example, 1 mL of drug may be dissolved in 10 mL of water or alcohol.

The label indicates whether the solution is a weight per volume (w/v) or volume per volume (v/v) type of solution by giving the units of measurement of the solute and the solvent.

1 tsp in 1 fluid oz is a volume per volume
1 g per 100 mL is a weight per volume

Medication labels indicate the strength of the drug available in solution. The strength may be stated as a percentage or as a ratio. For example, a 5% solution has 5 g of medication in every 100 mL of solution. If the label states: 1:1 000, this means that 1 g of drug is dissolved in 1 000 mL (or that the strength is 1 mg per mL). The amount of drug dissolved in solution may also be stated using other units of measure: examples include mmol, mEq, and U.

Exercise 4.2

Complete the following exercise without referring to the previous text. Correct using the answer guide. (Value: 1 each)

Complete each of the following sentences with the most appropriate term.

1. A homogeneous mixture that contains one or more dissolved substances in a liquid is called a _____ .

2. The substance that is dissolved in a solution is called a _____ .

3. In a solution, the liquid in which a substance is dissolved is called a _____ .

Read the label of this drug, then answer questions 4 and 5.

> Add 4.6 mL of sterile water to obtain
> penicillin G potassium 200 000 units per mL.

4.   In this drug solution, name the solute.

5.   In this drug solution, name the solvent.

Indicate whether the following sentence is true or false:

6.   The strength or concentration of a solution is determined by the amount of solute dissolved in a given amount of solvent.

For the following questions, choose the best answer.

7.   Which solution has the greater concentration?
     a. 1 000 units per 1 mL.
     b. 10 000 units per 1 mL.

8.   The labels on two vials of the same medication indicate that the concentrations are:
     Drug A: 10 mg/mL
     Drug B: 100 mg in 10 mL
     Is the concentration of Drug A:
         a. the same as that of Drug B?
         b. less than that of Drug B?
         c. greater than that of Drug B?

Complete questions 9 to 12 by indicating that unit of measurement for the solute and the solvent for each type of solution. Choose your response from this list of units: g, mg, or mL.

9.   In a weight per volume solution, the unit of measurement of the solute is a _____ .

10. In a weight per volume solution, the unit of measurement of the solvent is a _____ .

11. In a volume per volume solution, the unit of measurement of the solute is a _____ .

12. In a volume per volume solution, the unit of measurement of the solvent is a _____ .

In question 13 and 14, indicate whether the solutions are weight per volume or volume per volume:

13. A solution that has 5 g of solute, pure drug, dissolved in 100 mL of solvent is termed a _____ solution.

14. You have mixed 5 mL of lemon juice with 250 mL of water. You have prepared a _____ solution.

15. Drugs may be dissolved in liquid such as _____ .

Your Score: _____ **/15** = _____ %

Medication Labels

The medication label contains very important information. Some labels are clearly presented, provided your vision is satisfactory! Other labels are confusing. They are not standardized as to what information is included or how it is presented. It's important to develop the habit of thoroughly studying the information and instructions on drug labels. Accompanying literature also provides useful information. Check your habits: the last time you bought a piece of equipment — tape recorder, video machine, or pocket calculator — *did you read the instructions*?

The label below illustrated the type of information that should be included in drug packaging.

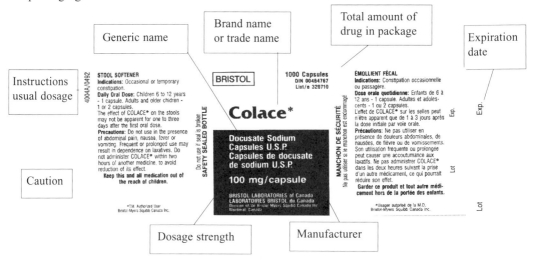

The brand or trade name is given by a manufacturer. The generic name is a brief form of the chemical name of the drug. The same generic drug may be sold under different brand or trade names. The same brand name may or may not be available in different countries. For example, the generic chlorpromazine is available as Thorazine in the U.S. and Largactil in Canada. It is important to learn both generic and trade names: sometimes the physician's order states one name and the label on the product gives the other!

NOTE: This book will not teach the drug names but uses actual names (both generic and trade) for you to practice reading labels and orders carefully.

Exercise 4.3

Complete the following exercise without referring to the previous text. Correct using the answer guide. (Value: 1 each)

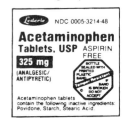

Refer to the label on the right and answer questions 1 to 3.

1. State the form of the drug.
2. What is the dosage strength?
3. State the drug name.

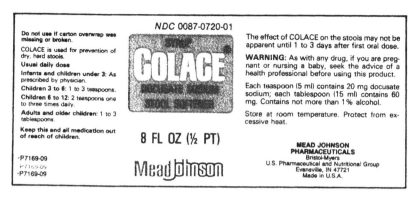

Refer to the above label and answer questions 4 to 10.

4. State the trade name of the drug.

5. State the generic name of the drug.

6. State the usual dose for adults. Convert the dose to mL.

7. What is the form of the drug?

8. What is the dosage strength of the drug?

9. What is the total volume contained in this bottle (in mL)?

10. If an adult took 2 tsp daily, how many days would the drug in this bottle last?

Your Score: _____ /10 = _____ %

Exercise 4.4

Complete the following exercise without referring to the previous pages. Correct using the answer guide. (Value: 1 each, unless otherwise indicated).

Interpret each of the following medication orders. Write out each of the underlined abbreviations in full.

1. Morphine sulfate 10–15 mg <u>IM q4h prn</u>

2. Insulin 6 units <u>SC stat</u>

3. Metoclopramide (Reglan) 10 mg <u>PO ac tid</u>

4. Aluminum hydroxide 30 mL <u>PO 1 h pc tid</u>

5. Flurazepam hydrochloride (Dalmane) 15 mg <u>PO hs</u>

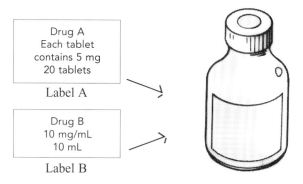

Label A

> Drug A
> Each tablet
> contains 5 mg
> 20 tablets

Label B

> Drug B
> 10 mg/mL
> 10 mL

Figure 4-4. Drug labels A and B

Refer to Figure 4-4 and answer questions 6 to 9.

	Label A	Label B
form of the drug	(6)	(7)
dosage strength	(8)	(9)

List the parts of a medication order. All medication orders should include the patient name, the drug name, the frequency or time of administration, the date, the physician's signature and the

10. d_____ ,

11. and r_____ .

12. A single-dose ampule labelled 25 mg/mL contains exactly 1 mL of liquid. True or false?

Match the abbreviation in column 1 with the correct expression in column 2.

Column 1

13. _____ pc
14. _____ stat.
15. _____ elix.
16. _____ ung.
17. _____ tab.
18. _____ ac
19. _____ cap.
20. _____ bid
21. _____ hs
22. _____ SC

Column 2

A. twice daily
B. capsule
C. ointment
D. at bedtime
E. after meals
F. elixir
G. immediately
H. tablet
I. before meals
J. subcutaneous

Read the label below and answer questions 23 to 30.

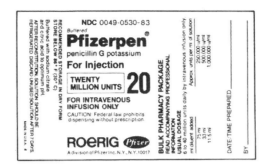

23. State the amounts of volume of diluent that may be added to the vial. (Value: 3)

24. What is the total amount of drug contained in this vial?

25. If 33 mL of diluent is added, what is the strength of the solution?

26. State the generic name of the drug.

27. State the trade name of the drug.

28. State the route of administration for the drug.

29. State the usual daily dosage range.

30. The solution is reconstituted on the fifteenth day of the month. When should unused solution be discarded?

Define each of the following terms in your own words and according to the module definitions. (Value: 2 each)

31. solute

32. solution

33. solvent

34. strength or concentration

Your Score: _____ **/40** = _____ **%**

Exercise 4.5

Complete the following to test your understanding of dosage forms and solutions. This information is essential for accurate dosage calculations. An example is done for you. (Value: 1 each)

Drug Product	Dosage Form	Concentration (per tablet or per mL)
furosemide (Lasix) single dose 4 mL vial containing 40 mg	* solution	* 10 mg per mL
furosemide (Lasix) oral solution 25 mL bottle containing 250 mg	(1)	(2)
125 mg	(3)	(4)
300 mg	(5)	(6)
haloperidol (Haldol) multidose vial = 5 mL containing 250 mg	(7)	(8)
1 mL ampule Haldol 5 mg	(9)	(10)
bottle of Stemetil prochlorperazine syrup; total volume in bottle is 100 mL total drug in bottle is 100 mg	(11)	(12)
Isoptin - 10 mg/4 mL (verapamil HCl)	(13)	(14)
HEP-LOCK	(15)	(16)
Dilantin	(17)	(18)
Kaon - Cl 20%	(19)	(20)

The label states ATROPINE 400 mcg/mL. State the amount of drug dissolved in each of the following volumes.

Volume	Drug Dose in mcg	Drug Dose in mg
2 mL	(21)	(22)
1.5 mL	(23)	(24)
1 mL	(25)	(26)
0.8 mL	(27)	(28)
0.5 mL	(29)	(30)

Your Score: _____ **/30** = _____ **%**

Exercise 4.6

Refer to the label and answer the questions. (Value: 1 each answer)

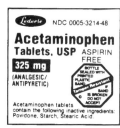

1. Drug name _____

2. Dosage form _____

3. Dosage strength _____

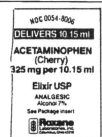

4. Drug name _____

5. Drug form _____

6. Dosage strength (per mL) _____
   Round to whole number.

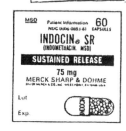

7. Brand or trade name _____

8. Generic name _____

9. Drug form _____

10. Dosage strength _____

11. Total number in package _____

12. Brand or Trade name _____

13. Generic name _____

14. Drug form _____

15. Dosage strength _____

16. Total number in package _____

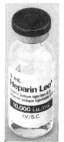

17. State the concentration of the lidocaine solution as a percent solution.

18. Explain what is meant by a 1% solution.

19. State the amount of lidocaine per mL of solution.

20. What is the total amount of lidocaine in the vial?

21. What is the total volume of lidocaine solution in the vial?

B

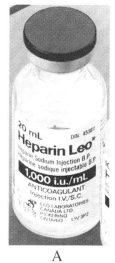

A

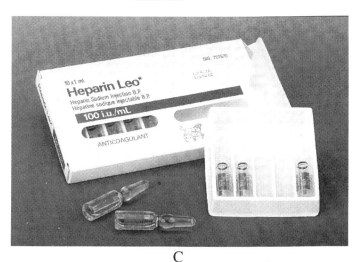

C

Refer to label A

22. What is the total amount of heparin sodium contained in this multi-dose vial?

23. What is the concentration of the heparin sodium solution? Name the solute in this solution.

24. What is the total volume contained in the vial?

Refer to label B

25. What is the concentration of the heparin sodium solution?

26. What is the total volume contained in the vial?

Refer to label C

27. What is the concentration of the heparin sodium solution?

28. What is the total volume contained in each ampule?

29. Compare the strengths of the solutions contained in the three heparin sodium products. Which product has the greatest concentration?

30. By what routes of administration can Heparin Leo be given?

Your Score: _____ /30 = _____ %

Optional Activity

Reading labels requires practice and attention. Learning where to find the information comes with experience. This book cannot provide enough situations, so you are encouraged to do any of the following activities to become familiar with drug product forms and labels.

1. Visit a drug store; browse; read labels and look for generic and trade names, the forms of the drugs, dosage strengths, number of tablets supplied, usual recommended doses, and other ingredients (e.g., preservatives, coloring).

2. Ask your clinical instructor or preceptor to show you various drug products in the clinical setting. Become familiar with the variety of labels and again look on each label for the name (generic and trade), other ingredients, drug form and strength, storage instructions, recommended dose, and administration precautions.

POSTTEST

Instructions

Write the posttest without referring to any reference materials.

Correct the posttest using the answer guide.

Part I

Complete the crossword with the abbreviations. (Value:21)

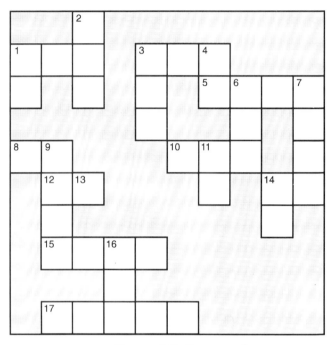

Figure 4-5. Crossword

Across

1. as required
2. unit
3. every 4 hours
5. immediately
8. after meals
10. twice daily
12. before meals
14. as much as is required
15. suspension
17. as desired, freely

Down

1. by mouth
2. ointment
3. four times a day
4. at bedtime
6. three times a day
7. tablets
9. capsule
11. intramuscular
14. with every hour
16. solution

Protect from light
Reconstitution:
Add Sterile Water for Injection according to the table below.
Shake Well. Use reconstituted stock solution within 8 hours.

Approx. Concentration	Amount of Diluent
200 mg/mL	45 mL
100 mg/mL	96 mL

Further dilute with one of the recommended I.V. solutions to a
desired concentration. Use further diluted solution within 24 hours
if kept at room temperature or 72 hours if refrigerated.
Usual Adult Dosage: 250 mg to 1 g every 6-12 hours.
See package insert. Monograph available on request.
Store dry powder at controlled room temperature below 25°C.

Date prepared
Prépare le _____

Diluent   Time
Solvant _____   Heure _____

                                 Prepared by
Concentration _____   Préparé par _____

DIN 01919628

⊞ANCEF®

STERILE CEFAZOLIN SODIUM USP
CÉFAZOLINE SODIQUE STÉRILE USP

10 g cefazolin/céfazoline

ANTIBIOTIC/ANTIBIOTIQUE

For Intravenous use / Pour usage intraveineux
Pharmacy bulk vial for single puncture, multiple dispensing
Fiole pour pharmacies, ponction unique, administrations multiples

SB SmithKline Beecham

Part II

Read the label above and answer questions 1 - 8. (Value: 1 each)

1. What is the form of the cefazolin sodium (Ancef)?

2. What is the route for administration?

3. What is the usual adult dose?

4. What is the suggested frequency for administration?

5. What diluent should be added?

6. How much diluent should be added to yield a solution of 100 mg/mL?

7. If 45 mL is added, what concentration is the solution?

8. What is the total amount of Ancef in this vial?

Part III

Write out the following orders. Do not use any abbreviations. (Value: 2 each)

1. Digoxin 250 mcg PO daily

2. Demerol 75 mg IM q 3-4h prn

3. Nitro spray SL prn

4. Nifedipine tab 20 mg PO bid

5. Nitroglycerin tab 0.3mg SL prn at bedside

6. Procainamide SR tab 750 mg PO tid

7. Glycerin supp PR prn

8. Salbutamol Inh 100 mcg/dose, 2 puffs q4-6 h

Part IV

Read the label and answer the questions. (Value: 5)

1. Name the solute in this drug preparation.

2. State the concentration of the solution.

3. State all the additives (preservatives) in

   this drug solution.

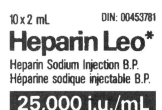

10 x 2 mL   DIN: 00453781

Heparin Leo*

Heparin Sodium Injection B.P.
Héparine sodique injectable B.P.

25,000 i.u./mL

ANTICOAGULANT
Injection I.V./S.C.

LEO LABORATORIES
CANADA LTD.
AJAX
L E O ONTARIO

*Regd. User Leo Laboratories Canada Ltd

Source: Intestinal Mucosa
Preservative Benzyl alcohol 1.0%
Methylparahydroxybenzoate 0.1%
Propylparahydroxybenzoate 0.02%
Average daily dose 20,000-40,000 units
1,000 units Heparin is neutralised by approx.
10 mg Protamine sulphate.
Store below 25°C
Full information available to practitioners
on request

Origine Muqueuse intestinale
Agent de conservation Alcool benzylique 1.0%
Parahydroxybenzoate de propyle 0.1%
Parahydroxybenzoate de methyle 0.02%
Posologie quotidienne moyenne
20 000-40 000 unités
Une dose de 1000 unités d'héparine est
neutralisée par environ 10 mg de sulfate
de protamine
À conserver au-dessous de 25°C
Information complète disponible aux
praticiens sur demande

Your Score: _____ **/50** = _____ **%**

100% **YES** — proceed to the next module

NO — review this module, rewrite the posttest, and obtain remedial
assistance if necessary.

Module 5: Calculation of Oral Medication Doses

Module Topics

- definitions
- calculating doses of tablets
- calculating doses of liquids
- case study & additional practice

Frequently, nurses must calculate and administer drugs or instruct patients and families in self-medication. Accurate calculation is extremely important for patient safety. This module describes how to calculate solid and liquid forms for oral administration, and provides practice exercises for the reader to develop an accurate and consistent approach. Clinical practice will further develop these skills.

CRITICAL POINT

Each time you administer a medication, check that you follow the five rights:

Right Drug:	read the medication order and the label
Right Dose:	calculate and validate
Right Route:	read the medication order and the label
Right Time:	read the medication order and the label
Right Patient:	read the medication order and the label

Some instructors might add 3 other "rights:"

Right Technique:	using aseptic procedures
Right Approach:	using interpersonal skills: e.g., explaining to a patient/family, calming a child before injection
Right Documentation:	accurately charting after administration according to the policy/records in the setting

---

Definitions

Please note that this book uses the following terms:

Dose: a portion of any therapeutic agent (drug) to be administered at one time. e.g., 325 mg of aspirin

Dosage: a system of doses: i.e. the dose and the frequency of interval of administration
e.g., aspirin 325 mg PO q4h

Strength or concentration: the available supply on hand stated as the amount of drug per tablet/capsule or the amount of drug dissolved in solution
e.g., 325 mg/tablet
e.g., 10 mg/mL

Calculating Doses of Tablets

The oral route is the most common for drug administration. Oral drug forms include solid forms such as tablets and capsules, and liquids such as elixirs, syrups, or suspensions.

Tablets or capsules contain a specific weight of a drug, commonly expressed in milligrams or grams. Liquid forms contain a specific amount of solute — medication — dissolved in a solvent (e.g., water or alcohol).

There are three methods for calculating solid drug forms.
A. Proportion using extremes and means
B. Proportion using cross product.
C. Formula

An example will illustrate each method. <u>You should decide which method you prefer and then use the same method consistently.</u>

Example: the order: diazepam 5 mg PO
Supply: available concentration diazepam (Valium) scored 10-mg tablets

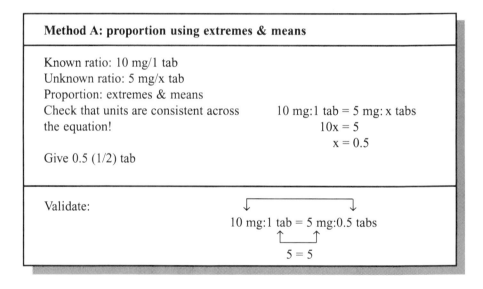

Method A: proportion using extremes & means

Known ratio: 10 mg/1 tab
Unknown ratio: 5 mg/x tab
Proportion: extremes & means
Check that units are consistent across   10 mg:1 tab = 5 mg: x tabs
the equation!   10x = 5
                                                              x = 0.5
Give 0.5 (1/2) tab

Validate:
                          10 mg:1 tab = 5 mg:0.5 tabs
                                       5 = 5

Method B: proportion using cross product

Known ratio: $\dfrac{10\ \text{mg}}{1\ \text{tab}}$

Unknown ratio: $\dfrac{5\ \text{mg}}{\text{x tab}}$

Proportion: cross product $\dfrac{10\ \text{mg}}{1\ \text{tab}} = \dfrac{5\ \text{mg}}{\text{x tab}}$

Check that units are consistent across
the equation!
Give 0.5 (1/2) tab

$$10x = 5$$
$$x = 0.5$$

Validate: $\dfrac{10\ \text{mg}}{1\ \text{tab}} = \dfrac{5\ \text{mg}}{0.5\ \text{tab}}$

$$5 = 5$$

CRITICAL POINT

When using proportion equations, be certain to check that the units
of measurement (e.g., mg, tabs, mL) are consistent across the equation. See
example below.

Example: the order is for a dose of 10 mg and the supply provides an available strength
of 5 mg tablets. Fill in the units in the following proportion equation:

5 _____ :1 _____ = 10 _____ :x _____

Solve the example using a formula. Several other nursing books use a variety of "formula statements" for calculation. These formula statements instruct that the dose is divided by
the available supply. For example:

Formula statement
$\dfrac{\text{dose (medication order)}}{\text{supply (available strength/concentration)}}$ = number of tablets/capsules

CRITICAL POINT

Relying on a "formula" presents some disadvantages. You might forget or misuse the formula. You cannot validate the answer with the formula but must use the proportion equation. Therefore, this book does not encourage this method.

Method C: formula

$$\frac{\text{dose}}{\text{supply}} = \frac{5 \text{ mg}}{10 \text{ mg}}$$

Give 0.5 (1/2) tab

Validate: use cross product	$\dfrac{10 \text{ mg}}{1 \text{ tab}} = \dfrac{5 \text{ mg}}{0.5 \text{ tab}}$
	$5 = 5$

CRITICAL POINT

Throughout this book, you will be asked to calculate a specific dose by using the available supply (strength or concentration) of a drug product. You must always state the answer in full; i.e., including tabs/caps or mL.

Some calculations look "easy" and you can "see" the answer immediately. Always check your answer intuitively: does it make sense? However, you should also develop a thorough and careful approach to calculations: develop the habit of validating your answer. Calculate — then validate!

Exercise 5.1

Complete the following exercise and correct using the Answer Guide. Calculate the dose then validate. State the answer in full (including tabs or caps). (Value: 3 for each question, 1 for correct calculation, 1 for validation, and 1 for including correct unit in answer)

1.   Order: theophylline 450 mg PO pc
Supply: theophylline (Theo-Dur) 300 mg scored tabs
Calculate:
Validate:

2.   Order: bromocriptine mesylate 5 mg PO daily
Supply: bromocriptine mesylate (Parlodel) 2.5 mg tablets
Calculate:
Validate:

3.   Order: nadolol 40 mg PO hs
Supply: nadolol (Corgard) 80 mg scored tablets
Calculate:
Validate:

4.   Order: meperidine 75 mg PO for pain
Supply: meperidine (Demerol) 50 mg scored tablets
Calculate:
Validate:

5.   Order: hydrochlorothiazide 100 mg PO daily
Supply: hydrochlorothiazide (HydroDiuril) 50 mg tablets
Calculate:
Validate:

6.   Order: Drug A 30 mg PO stat
Supply: two bottles labelled: Drug A 5 mg tablets and Drug A 20 mg tablets. Be sure to state which strength you are using and how many tablets to administer. Tabs are not scored.
Calculate:
Validate:

7.   Order: digoxin 0.125 mg PO daily
Supply: digoxin (Lanoxin) 0.25 mg scored tablets
Calculate:
Validate:

8.   Order: levothyroxine sodium 0.1 mg PO daily
Supply: levothyroxine sodium (Eltroxin) 0.05 mg tablets
Calculate:
Validate:

9. Order: Drug B 0.05 mg
Supply: scored tablets 0.1 mg
Calculate:
Validate:

10. Order: aspirin 650 mg PO
Supply: aspirin 325 mg tablets
Calculate:
Validate:

Your Score: _____ /30 = _____ %

Sometimes, the dose and the supply on hand are in different units of measurement. In these situations, you must convert and express the dose and the available strength/concentration in the same units. Recall the conversions you made in module 3. Study the following example and then proceed to the exercise for practice.

Example: Order for dose of 1.5 g. The supply on hand is 500 mg capsules.
Step 1: state dose in mg
Convert: 1.5 g = 1 500 mg (Recall: 1 g = 1 000 mg)
Calculate: cross product method

$$\frac{500 \text{ mg}}{1 \text{ cap}} = \frac{1\,500 \text{ mg}}{x \text{ caps}}$$

Note that the units are the same on both sides of the equation: cancel the units and solve.
500 x = 1 500
x = 3
Give 3 caps

Validate: proportion extremes & means
500 mg: 1 cap = 1 500 mg: 3 caps
Multiply extremes: 500 × 3 = 1 500
Multiply means: 1 × 1 500 = 1 500
1 500 = 1 500

Exercise 5.2

Calculate the following dosages. (Value: 2 each; 1 for correct conversion and 1 for correct answer). Be careful to include the appropriate unit of measure with your answer; e.g., tablet, mg, mL.

1. Order: 0.015 g of Drug B
   Label: 5 mg tablets
   Give: _____

2. Order: 1.5 g PO tid
   Label: 500 mg tablets
   Give: _____

3. Order: 0.2 g prn
   Label: 100 mg tablets
   Give: _____

4. Order: 1 g stat
   Label: 250 mg tablets
   Give: _____

5. Order: 1 g q6h
   Label: 500 mg tablets
   Give: _____

6. Order: 0.5 g qid
   Label: 250 mg capsules
   Give: _____

7. Order: 0.15 mg PO daily
   Label: 0.05 mg tablets
   Give: _____

8. Order: 0.125 mg PO q am
   Label: 125 mcg tablets
   Give: _____

9. Order: 500 mg qid × 3 weeks
   Label: 250 mg capsules
   How many capsules will be required for a 3-week supply? _____

10. Order: digoxin 0.125 mg PO daily
    Label: digoxin (Lanoxin) 125 mcg tablets
    Give: _____

Your Score: _____ /20 = _____ %

Exercise 5.3: Practice Reading Labels

Refer to the labels on page 77 to solve the following problems. For each order, state the correct amount to administer to provide the ordered dose. Be sure to state the strength of the available supply as indicated on the label. (Value: 1 each answer)

CRITICAL POINT

There are many types of medication supply systems. The labels used in each system differ greatly, and you need to practice locating important information. For safety and accuracy, read the label three times; once as you select the product/package, again as you calculate/confirm the dose, and finally as you replace/discard the package.

---

1. Order: phenobarbital 15 mg PO bid
   (a) strength:
   (b) calculation:

2. Order: Baclofen 10 mg PO tid
   (a) strength:
   (b) calculation:

3. Order: docusate sodium 200 mg hs
   (a) strength:
   (b) calculation:

4. Dose is phenobarbital 15 mg PO in am and 30 mg PO hs
   (a) strength:
   (b) calculate am dose:
   (c) strength:
   (d) calculate hs dose:

5. Dose of Lanoxin 0.25 mg PO daily
   (a) strength:
   (b) calculation:

6. A woman accidentally took 2 tablets of her digoxin (0.125 mg strength). How many mcg did she ingest?

7. Dose of Baclofen 15 mg tid × 4 days then 10 mg tid × 3 days.
   (a) strength and calculation for initial dose:
   (b) strength and calculation for second dose:
   (c) required supply for 7 days:

8. A child swallowed all of the 20 mg Lioresal. How much was ingested?

9. Order states phenobarbital 30 mg PO bid and 45 mg PO hs
   (a) strength and calculation for daytime doses:
   (b) strength and calculation for bedtime dose:
   (c) total daily dose:

Your Score: _____ /20 = _____ %

Use these drug labels to answer Exercise 5.3. Practice reading the label three times!

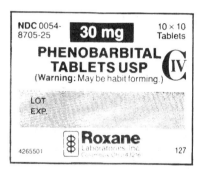

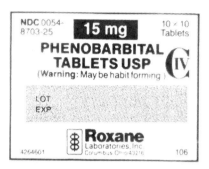

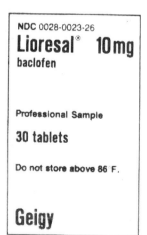

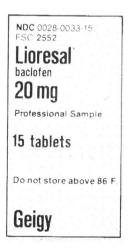

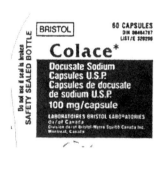

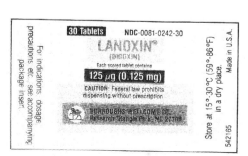

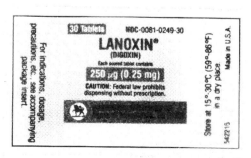

Exercise 5.4: Additional Practice

Complete then correct using the Answer Guide. (Value: 1 each answer)

1. Order: ampicillin 500 mg PO bid
Available: 250 mg caps of ampicillin (Novo-Ampicillin)
(a) Number of caps for each dose:
(b) Number of caps required for one day supply:

2. Order: allopurinol 300 mg PO daily
Available: allopurinol (Zyloprim) 100 mg tabs
(a) Number of tabs for each dose:
(b) Number of tabs required for one day supply:

3. Order: cephalexin 1 g PO q6h
Available: cephalexin (Keflex) 500 mg tabs
(a) Number of tabs for each dose:
(b) Number of tabs required for one day supply:

4. Order: levothyroxine sodium 0.15 mg PO daily
Available: levothyroxine sodium (Synthroid) 0.05 mg tabs
(a) Number of tabs for each dose:
(b) Number of tabs required for one day supply:

5. Order: theophylline 450 mg PO pc
Available: theophylline (Theo-Dur) 300 mg scored tabs
(a) Number of tabs for each dose:
(b) Number of tabs required for one day supply:

6. Order: digoxin 125 mcg PO q am
Available: digoxin (Lanoxin) 0.125 mg tabs
(a) Number of tabs for each dose:
(b) Number of tabs required for one day supply:

7. Order: penicillin G potassium 1 000 000 units PO qid
Available: tablets labelled 500 000 units
(a) Number of tabs for each dose:
(b) Number of tabs required for one day supply:

8. Order: aspirin 0.65 g PO q6h
Available: aspirin 325 mg tabs
(a) Number of tabs for each dose:
(b) Number of tabs required for one day supply:

9. Order: captopril 0.05 g PO bid
Available: captopril (Capoten) 25 mg tabs
(a) Number of tabs for each dose:
(b) Number of tabs required for one day supply:

10. Order: sulfasalazine 1 g PO qid
Available: 500 mg tabs
(a) Number of tabs for each dose:
(b) Number of tabs required for one day supply:

Your Score: _____ /20 = _____ %

Calculating Doses of Liquids

Medications may be administered orally in suspensions and solutions. You should learn the following definitions:

Solution: one or more drugs dissolved in a liquid

Suspension: fine particles of a drug are suspended in a liquid base; appears cloudy; shake well before using: includes emulsions, magmas, and gels

Elixir: aromatic, sweetened solution containing a dissolved medication; has various percentages of alcohol

Calculation of liquid forms should be done using proportion (either extremes & means or cross product, as you prefer).

NOTE: Although some references use a formula statement, it is not recommended, as it has a greater risk of error in calculation.

CRITICAL POINT

Oral liquid medications are often poured into a one-ounce measuring cup. When measuring liquid in this container, it is important to view the curve of the liquid, called the meniscus, at eye level. You should read the bottom of the curve, as illustrated in Figure 5.1.

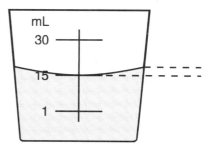

Figure 5.1 Reading a meniscus. A meniscus is caused by the surface tension of a solution against container walls. The surface tension causes the formation of a concave or hollowed curvature on the solution surface. Read the level at the lowest point of concave curve.

Review the sample problem and then proceed to Exercise 5.5 for practice calculating oral liquid doses.

Problem: The order is for thioridazine hydrochloride 60 mg PO prn and the available concentration is thioridazine hydrochloride (Mellaril) 25 mg/5 mL.

Method A: proportion using extremes & means

Known ratio: 25 mg/5 mL
Unknown ratio: 60 mg/x tab
Proportion: extremes & means
Check that units are consistent across   25 mg:5 mL = 60 mg: x mL
the equation!   25 x = 300
                                                                        x = 12

Give 12 mL to provide the dose of 60 mg

Validate:

$$25 \text{ mg: } 5 \text{ mL} = 60 \text{ mg:} 12 \text{ mL}$$
$$25 \times 12 = 300$$
$$5 \times 60 = 300$$

Method B: proportion using cross product

Known ratio: $\dfrac{25 \text{ mg}}{5 \text{ mL}}$

Unknown ratio: $\dfrac{60 \text{ mg}}{x \text{ mL}}$

Proportion: cross product $\dfrac{25 \text{ mg}}{5 \text{ mL}} = \dfrac{60 \text{ mg}}{x \text{ mL}}$

Check that units are consistent across $25x = 300$
the equation! $x = 12$
Give 12 mL to provide dose of 60 mg

Validate: $\dfrac{25 \text{ mg}}{5 \text{ mL}} = \dfrac{60 \text{ g}}{12 \text{ mL}}$
                              $(25 \times 12) = (5 \times 60)$
                                    $300 = 300$

Exercise 5.5

Complete the exercise without referring to the previous text. If you have difficulty doing conversions between the household and metric systems, review Table 3-4. Correct using the Answer Guide. (Value: 1 each answer)

CRITICAL POINT

Dosage errors often result from carelessness. Whenever you calculate a dosage, check the answer to see if it seems reasonable.

Refer to the labels on page 82 and answer questions 1 to 20.

State the total volume, in mL, in each drug container.

1. Colace oral solution   _____ mL
2. Pen-Vee K oral solution   _____ mL
3. Kaon-Cl   _____ mL
4. Benadryl elixir   _____ mL
5. Dilantin suspension   _____ mL

For each order, state the volume to be administered.

6. Benadryl 12.5 mg. How many mL?
7. Benadryl 12.5 mg. How many tsp?
8. Benadryl 25 mg. How many mL?
9. Dilantin 100 mg. How many mL?
10. Phenytoin 125 mg. How many tsp?
11. Potassium chloride 20 mEq. How many mL?
12. Pen-Vee K 200 000 units. How many mL?
13. Pen-Vee K 200 mg. How many mL?
14. Pen-Vee K 400 000 units. How many tsp?
15. Colace 100 mg. How many mL?

For each of the following orders, refer to the labels on page 81. Calculate the total number of doses that can be given from the volume indicated on the drug label.

16. Dilantin 125 mg PO tid
17. Diphenhydramine 50 mg PO bid
18. Penicillin V Potassium 400 000 units PO tid
19. Docusate sodium 100 mg PO
20. Potassium chloride 40 mEq PO daily

Your Score: _____ /20 = _____ %

Refer to these labels to work on questions 16–20 in Exercise 5.5.

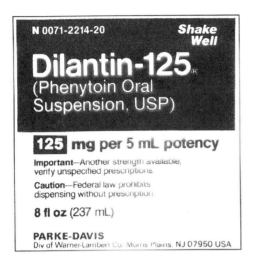

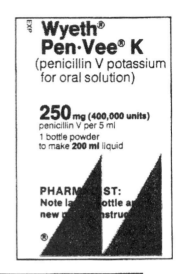

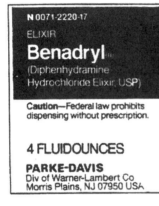

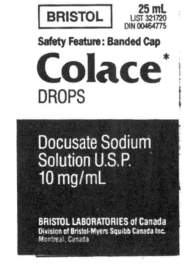

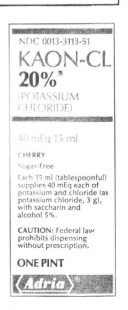

Exercise 5.6: Finding Errors

This activity is designed to help you develop a consistent and accurate approach to setting up the problem before you calculate the answer. Each of the following problems and calculations has an error. Find the error and determine the correct calculation.

1. Order: phenobarbital 0.3 g PO. Strength on hand: tablets labelled 100 mg
Calculate: convert dose to mg: $0.3 \text{ g} = x \text{ mg} = 3\,000 \text{ mg}$

Proportion: cross product: $\dfrac{100 \text{ mg}}{1 \text{ tab}} = \dfrac{3\,000 \text{ mg}}{x \text{ tabs}}$

$$100 \text{ x} = 3\,000$$
$$x = 30$$

Give 30 tabs? Does this make sense? Find the error.

2. Order: warfarin 5 mg PO. Strength on hand: tablets labelled 2.5 mg. Calculate using the formula: $\dfrac{2.5 \text{ mg}}{5 \text{ mg}} = 0.5 \text{ tab}$

Give 0.5 tab? There is always a risk using any formula: it is easy to "forget" the formula. Find the solution using proportion.

3. From tablets labelled "1 gram" give a dose of 2 500 mg.
Calculation: $1:1 \text{ tab} = 2\,500:x \text{ tabs}$
$$x = 2\,500$$
Obviously, there is a serious error here: you cannot possibly give 2 500 tabs. What is wrong?

4. Order: 30 mg of an elixir. Strength (or concentration) on hand is labelled "15 mg per 5 mL"
Calculation: $5:15 = 30:x$
$$5x = 450$$
$$x = 90$$
Give 90 mL. What is wrong?

5. Give a dose of digoxin 0.125 mg from tablets labelled 0.25 mg
Answer: give 5 tabs.
Too often, the nurse might "see" the answer without carefully writing out the problem. This error actually does occur in the clinical setting (and is very serious). Find the correct answer.

Additional Practice

> ### CASE STUDY
>
> Mr. B., a 79-year-old man, is admitted to an acute care hospital with congestive heart failure. Medication orders include:
>
> Lasix 80 mg PO today then 40 mg daily
> digoxin 0.375 mg today only
> digoxin 0.25 mg PO starting tomorrow
> levothyroxine sodium 0.075 mg daily

Refer to the Medication Cupboard in Figure 5.2 on page 86.

1. State the generic and trade name of each product. (Value: 6)

2. State the available strengths for each of the following drugs. (Value: 12)
   Lanoxin
   Lasix
   Synthroid
   Eltroxin

3. Calculate all doses for today for Mr. B. State which product you are using and number of tablets to give. (Value: 6)

Product	Number of Tablets to Give
1.	2.
3.	4.
5.	6.

4. Calculate all doses for tomorrow for Mr. B. State which product you are using. and number of tablets to give. (Value: 6)

Product	Number of Tablets to Give
1.	2.
3.	4.
5.	6.

5. Arrange the strengths of Synthroid from the greatest (highest dose) to the least. (Value: 1)

6. Calculate doses for the am administration of omeprazole for the following 3 days. (Value: 3)
   Day 1: 60 mg PO q am
   Day 2: 80 mg PO q am
   Day 3: 60 mg PO q am and 60 mg PO at hs

7. Give Lozide 2.5 mg PO. (Value: 1)

8. The order is for levothyroxine sodium 0.3 mg. Which product will you use and why? (Value: 1)

9. If 0.05 mg of levothyroxine sodium is ordered, calculate all possible choices of products and amounts to give. Assume tabs are <u>not</u> scored; whole tabs must be used. State which products and strengths would be most desirable to use. (Value: 4)

10. If 1 tablet of each product of digoxin is given what would be the total dosage? (Value: 1)

11. State the strength of all Lanoxin products in micrograms (mcg). (Value: 3)

12. Calculate all possible combinations of products to give 80 mg of furosemide. (Value: 3) Example: give 1 × 80 mg tablet

13. Calculate: order Synthroid 100 mcg PO. (Value: 1)

14. Calculate: order digoxin 125 mcg PO. (Value: 1)

15. Calculate: order omeprazole 20 mg PO. (Value: 1)

Your Score: _____ **/50** = _____ **%**

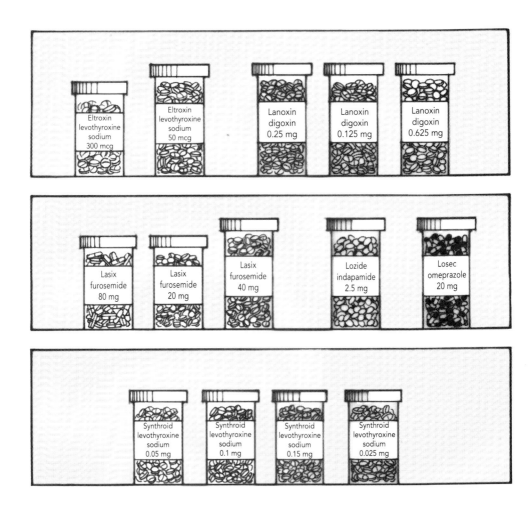

Figure 5.2. Medication Cupboard

POSTTEST

Instructions

Write the posttest without referring to any reference materials

Correct using the answer guide

Be careful to include all units with the answer (e.g., mg, mL, tabs.)

Round decimal numbers to the nearest whole number

Validate all answers

(Value: 3 each; 1 for correct calculation, 1 for correct unit, 1 for validation)

1. The order is: phenobarbital 0.3 g PO. The strength on hand is 100 mg tablets.
2. The order is glyburide 1.25 mg PO. The strength on hand is 2.5 mg scored tablets.
3. From warfarin tablets of 2.5 mg each, calculate for an order of 2.5 mg on even days and 5 mg on odd days: Use today's date.
4. Aspirin 0.65 g is ordered. You have tablets of 325 mg each.
5. The patient is to receive 0.8 mg of drug S. The label states 0.4 mg/tab.
6. The physician orders 0.125 mg of digoxin PO. daily. The drug is labelled 125 mcg/tab. How many tablets would the patient require for a 2 week supply?
7. You are to give 2 500 mg of drug B. The label indicates that each tablet is 1 g.
8. The order states 75 mg PO prn for pain. The strength on hand is 50 mg scored tablets.
9. The patient is to receive 35 mg of an elixir. The bottle in the drug cabinet reads 15 mg/5 mL. If 12 mL was administered, what dose did the patient actually receive?
10. The order is for 500 mg q6h. The drug label reads 250 mg/5 mL.

Refer to the labels below and answer questions 11 to 20.

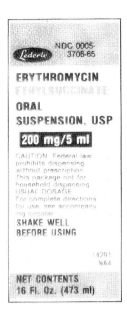

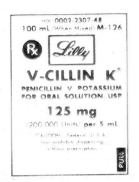

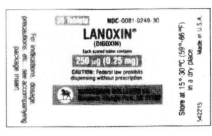

11. Give erythromycin 150 mg PO.

12. A mother gave her child 1 tsp of erythromycin. What dosage of drug did the child receive?

13. Give erythromycin 75 mg PO.

14. Give digoxin 0.125 mg PO.

15. Give 100 mg V-cillin K PO.

16. Read the V-cillin label. How many units comprise 1 mg?

17. Give 125 000 units of V-cillin K PO.

18. Read the Lanoxin label. How many mcg are contained in 1.5 tabs?

19. What is the total amount of penicillin V potassium in mg and units in the bottle?

20. How many units of drug are there per mL of penicillin V potassium oral solution in the bottle?

Your Score: _____ /60 = _____ %

100% **YES** — proceed to the next module

NO — review this module

Module 6: Calculation of Parenteral Medication Doses

Module Topics

- reading calibrated medication equipment
- calculating parenteral medications
- reconstituting medication doses
- additional practice
- case study

Administration of medications by the parenteral route (SC, IM, or IV) requires greater precision than the oral route. Whereas you might give a teaspoon of oral liquid (which is approximately 5 mL) you will calculate and give parenteral doses such as 0.4 mL and 1.25 mL.

CRITICAL POINT

It is safe clinical practice to always calculate parenteral doses on paper and to validate your work. In some clinical settings, it is a requirement to double-check the dose with a colleague. Know the policies of each setting.

This module will provide the opportunity to develop and practice skills of calculation of common doses. More complex situations (e.g., mixing two medications in one syringe) are described in Module 8.

Reading Calibrated Medication Equipment

Before studying the calculation of liquid medications for parenteral administration, you should be familiar with the calibration of syringes. This module does not acquaint you with the procedure of injections. Examine the figures only to become familiar with the calibration of each type of syringe.

Figure 6.1 Syringes

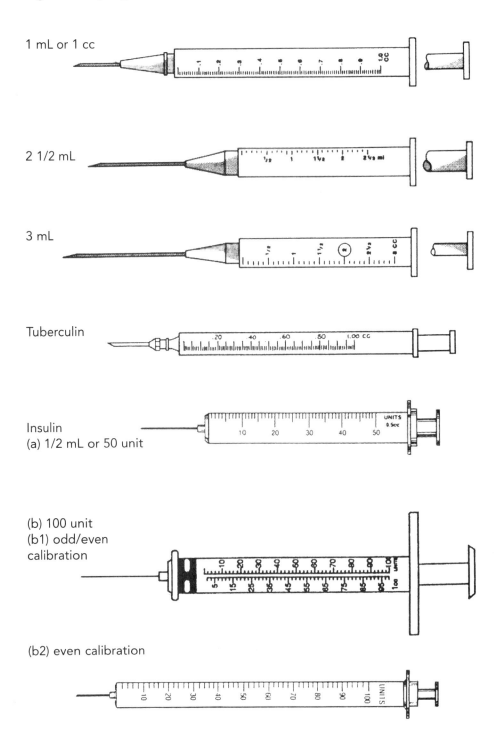

1 mL or 1 cc

2 1/2 mL

3 mL

Tuberculin

Insulin
(a) 1/2 mL or 50 unit

(b) 100 unit
(b1) odd/even
calibration

(b2) even calibration

Exercise 6.1

For each syringe, state (a) the total volume of the syringe and (b) the volume indicated by the shading. (Value: 2 each) An example is done for you.

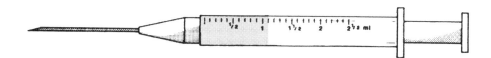

Example: (a) total volume of syringe 2 1/2 mL (b) volume of liquid 1.1 mL

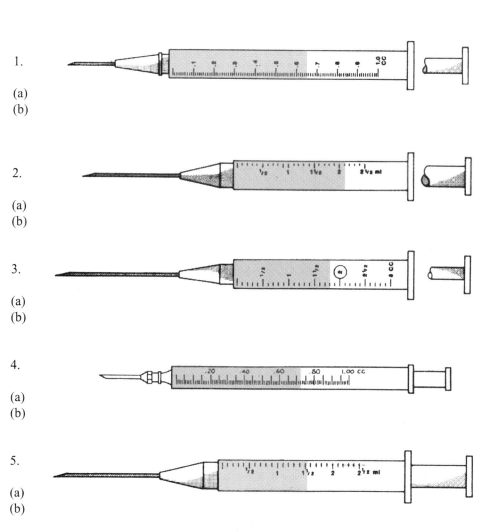

1.
(a)
(b)

2.
(a)
(b)

3.
(a)
(b)

4.
(a)
(b)

5.
(a)
(b)

Your Score: _____ **/10** = _____ **%**

Calculating Parenteral Medication Doses

Once again, there are different approaches to calculating doses of parenteral liquid medications. You should use the same method consistently and always validate your answer.

Method A: ratio and proportion: extremes × means
Method B: ratio and proportion: cross-product method
Method C: formula

Problem: give 75 mg IM using a 2 mL ampule labeled "50 mg/mL".

Solve with ratio and proportion.

METHOD A: Extremes × means	**METHOD B: Cross Product**
known ratio: 50 mg in 1 mL unknown ratio: 75 mg in x mL multiple extremes and means 50:1 = 75:x 50 x = 75 x = 75/50 = 1.5 Give 1.5 mL	known ratio: 50 mg/1 mL unknown ratio: 75 mg/x mL cross-product multiplication $\frac{50}{1}$ ⤬ $\frac{75}{x}$ 50 x = 75 $x = \frac{75}{50}$ x = 1.5 Give 1.5 mL
Validate: 50:1 = 75:1.5 50 × 1.5 = 1 × 75 75 = 75	Validate: 50/1 = 75/1.5 75 = 75

METHOD C: Solve using the formula.

$$\frac{\text{dose}}{\text{supply}} \times \text{volume} = \text{amount to administer}$$

METHOD C: Formula

$$\frac{\text{dose}}{\text{supply}} \times \text{volume} = \text{amount to administer}$$

$$\frac{75 \text{ mg}}{50 \text{ mg}} \times 1 \text{ mL} = \text{x mL}$$

x = 1.5
give 1.5 mL

Always include the units to ensure you have set up the formula correctly. There are disadvantages to using the formula method. First, you may forget the formula or you may insert the values into the formula incorrectly. Second, it is difficult to validate the answer: ratio and proportion must be used for validation.

Check your answer "intuitively." A 2 mL ampule contains 100 mg of drug (50 mg per mL). To give 75 mg, you have calculated 1.5 mL. Does it seem right?

Exercise 6.2

Complete the following exercise without referring to the previous text. Correct using the answer guide. Be careful that the appropriate units are part of your answer, e.g., mg, mL. Include two places to the right of the decimal (hundredths) in your response. (Value: Q 1-6; 2 each, 1 for calculation, 1 for correct unit)

1. The order is: heparin 7 500 units SC. You have a 5 mL vial of heparin labeled: 10 000 units/mL. Determine the correct dosage to administer.

2. The label on a 2 mL ampule indicates 50 mg/mL. How many mg are contained in 1.5 mL?

3. The vial label states: 250 mg ampicillin per mL. Calculate 400 mg IM.

4. Your patient has an order for meperidine (Demerol) 75 mg IM. The 2 mL ampule is labeled: 50 mg/mL. How many mL should the patient receive?

5. The drug label states: 100 mg/mL. Calculate 80 mg dose.

6. The antibiotic label states: 400 000 units/mL. If 1 mg = 1 600 units calculate a dose of 200 mg.

For each of the following questions, <u>shade</u> in the accompanying syringe to indicate the correct dosage. (Value: 2 each; 1 for calculation, 1 for correct shading)

7. Ordered: heparin 5 000 units SC
   On hand: heparin 10 000 units/mL

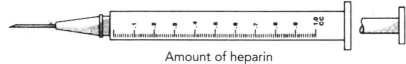

Amount of heparin

Dosage Calculations in SI Units

8. Ordered: morphine 12 mg IM
   On hand: morphine 15 mg/mL

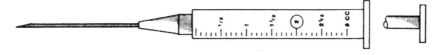

Amount of morphine and perphenazine

9. Ordered: dimenhydrinate (Gravol) 30 mg IM prn
   On hand: dimenhydrinate 50 mg/mL

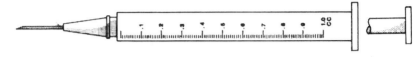

Amount of dimenhydrinate

10. An analgesic is ordered: 75 mg IM stat. On hand is a 2-mL ampule with a dosage concentration of 50 mg/mL. Calculate the dose to administer.

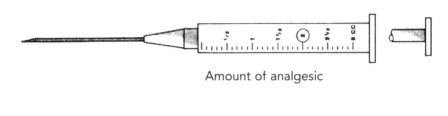

Amount of analgesic

Your Score: _____ /20 = _____ %

Exercise 6.3

Read the amount (volume) of medication in each of these syringes.

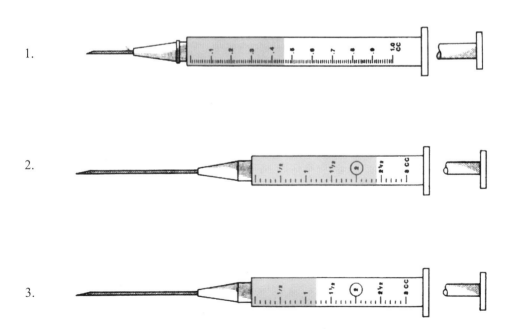

1.

2.

3.

4.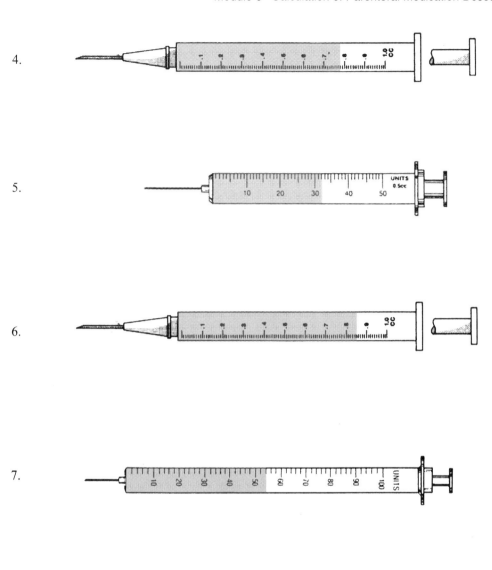

5.

6.

7.

8.

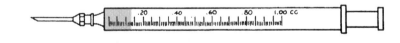

Your Score: _____ **/8** = _____ **%**

Reconstituting Medications

To increase their stability, some medications are prepared in a dry powder form and must be diluted with a sterile solvent before administration. For example, many antibiotics must be reconstituted with sterile water. Refer to Table 6-1, which illustrates a dilution table on a multiple-dose vial. Note that adding 46 mL of sterile diluent yields a solution with 200 000 IU (International Units) of medication in each millilitre. Contrast this concentration with the solution that results when only 6 mL of diluent, usually sterile water, are added.

Table 6-1. Reconstitution of a Powdered Drug

Potency Required IU per mL	Add Sterile Aqueous Diluent
200 000	46 mL
250 000	36 mL
750 000	9.3 mL
1 000 000	6 mL

CRITICAL POINT

When a certain volume of liquid is added to a powdered drug in a vial, the resulting product will usually be of a greater volume. For example, adding 9.3 mL of fluid may result in a final volume in the vial of 10 mL. The powdered drug occupies some volume.

When preparing a liquid from a powder form:

1. Read directions on the label or package insert.
2. Select the diluent (the label will state at least one of):
   • sterile water for injection
   • bacteriostatic water (has a preservative)
   • normal saline for injection.
3. Decide what concentration to prepare, based on required dose and route of administration.
4. Inject air into vial of diluent to create positive pressure, and withdraw desired amount of diluent.
5. A. Inject the diluent into vial of powdered drug. B. Shake well to produce a homogenous mixture.
6. Date and initial the vial: indicate the amount of diluent added.
7. Calculate and withdraw the correct amount for the required dose.
8. Store the vial according to directions.

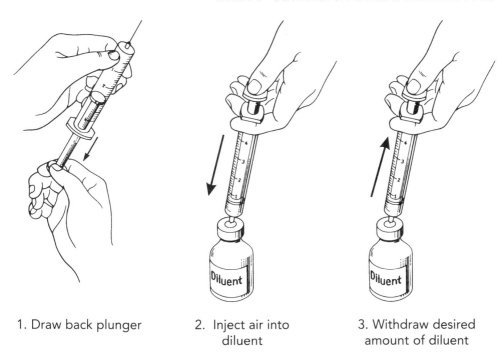

1. Draw back plunger

2. Inject air into diluent

3. Withdraw desired amount of diluent

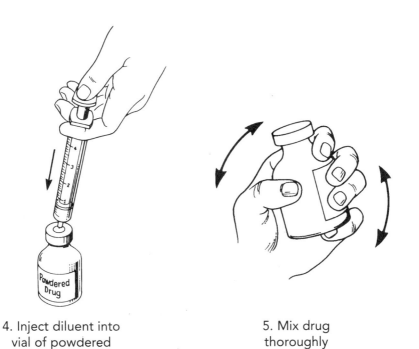

4. Inject diluent into vial of powdered medication

5. Mix drug thoroughly

Figure 6-2 illustrates the reconstitution of a powdered drug form. Study the figure and the following example, and proceed to the exercise.

Example:

Vial of penicillin G potassium contains 5 million units of drug. Package instructions specify "sterile water for injection." Directions are:

Volume of diluent to be added (mL)	Approximate available volume (mL)	Approximate concentrations (potency) (IU/mL)
3	5	1 000 000
8	10	500 000
18	20	250 000

Write directly on label of the vial.
For example, to give a dose of 250 000 IU, add 18 mL, shake well to mix evenly, and withdraw 1 mL.

Although reconstituted drugs may be stored at room temperature, they remain stable for longer periods in the refrigerator. Practice reading labels in the clinical situation to become familiar with this technique.

PROBLEM: give penicillin G potassium 400 000 units IM q4h

1. Read label

2. Add diluent: choose 4.6 mL

3. State dosage strength
   200 000 units/mL

4. Calculate
   Known: 200 000 units:1 mL
   Unknown: 400 000 units : x mL
   200 000:1 = 400 000: x
   200 000 x = 400 000
   x = 2
   answer: 2 mL

5. Validate
   $$\frac{200\ 000}{1} = \frac{400\ 000}{2}$$

6. Circle the dosage strength prepared, date and initial the label.

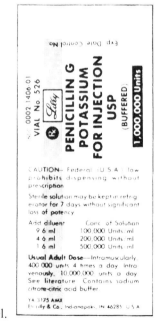

Exercise 6.4

Answer and check with the answer guide. Refer to this label to answer questions 1-8. Round to nearest tenth. (Value: 1 each)

Potency Required IU per mL	Add Sterile Aqueous Diluent
200 000	46 mL
250 000	36 mL
750 000	9.3 mL
1 000 000	6 mL

1. The order is for 750 000 units IM q4h. How much diluent would you add to yield a solution with a concentration of 750 000 units/mL?

2. The medication has been mixed by another nurse and the vial is signed, dated, and marked to indicate that 9.3 mL of sterile diluent was added. How much would be required to administer a dose of 1 million units?

You add 46 mL of sterile diluent and mix the powdered drug. For each of the following orders, indicate the correct volume to administer:

3. 750 000 units

4. 400 000 units

5. 250 000 units

You add 36 mL of sterile diluent and mix the powdered drug. For each of the following volumes, indicate the amount of drug (in units):

6. 1 mL

7. 0.8 mL

8. 1.4 mL

Read the Ampicin label and answer questions 9-12.

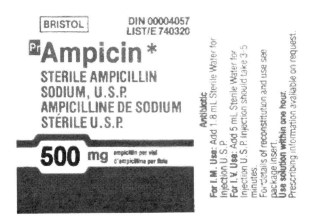

9. State the volume and type of diluent to be added for IM use.

10. How long is reconstituted solution stable?

11. Calculate the volume to administer 500 mg. (Note: final volume after adding diluent is 2 mL)

12 What is the generic name?

Read the Cefizox label and answer questions 13-17.

13. State the generic name.

14. State the volume and type of diluent for IM use.

15. State the resulting concentration.

16. How long is the reconstituted solution stable?

17. Calculate volume for 500 mg IM.

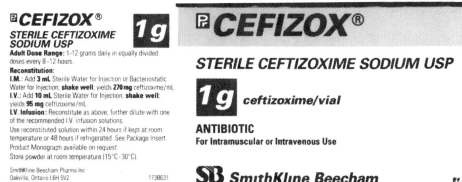

Read the Ancef label and answer questions 18-20.

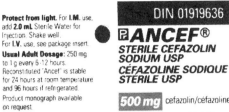

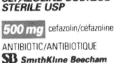

DIN 01919636

⊞ANCEF®
STERILE CEFAZOLIN
SODIUM USP
CÉFAZOLINE SODIQUE
STERILE USP

500 mg cefazolin/céfazoline

ANTIBIOTIC/ANTIBIOTIQUE
SB *SmithKline Beecham*

Protect from light. For I.M. use, add **2.0 mL** Sterile Water for Injection. Shake well. For **I.V.** use, see package insert. **Usual Adult Dosage:** 250 mg to 1 g every 6-12 hours. Reconstituted 'Ancef' is stable for 24 hours at room temperature and 96 hours if refrigerated. Product monograph available on request

SmithKline Beecham Pharma Inc. Oakville, Ontario L6H 5V2

Craint la lumière. Pour usage **i.m.,** ajouter **2,0 mL** d'eau stérile pour injection. Bien agiter. Pour usage **i.v.,** voir notice. **Posologie habituelle pour adultes :** 250 mg à 1 g toutes les 6 à 12 heures. Remis en solution, 'Ancef' est stable pendant 24 heures à la température ambiante et pendant 96 heures sous réfrigération. Monographie sur demande. Can. Lic. No. 147

173H941

18. State the volume and type of diluent, for IM use.

19. If resulting concentration is 225 mg/mL, calculate the volume for a dose of 250 mg IM.

20. Calculate the volume for a dose of 400 mg IM.

Your Score: _____ /20 = _____ %

Exercise 6.5

For further practice, calculate the following dosages: (Value 2: each; 1 for calculation, and 1 for correct unit)

NOTE: be careful to include the appropriate unit of measure with your answer, e.g., tablet, mg, mL. Round decimal numbers to the nearest hundredth.

1. The order is for 8 000 units IV stat. The vial is labeled 10 000 units/mL. Determine the correct dose.

2. The penicillin vial is labeled 200 000 units/mL. The order is 80 000 units IM. Determine the correct dose.

3. The order is perphenazine 3.5 mg IM stat. The ampule is labeled 5 mg/mL. Determine the correct volume to administer.

4. From hydrocortisone 100 mg/2 mL, determine the correct dosage for 75 mg IM daily.

5. The order is meperidine 75 mg IM prn. The ampule is labeled meperidine 100 mg/mL. Determine the correct dosage.

6. You must administer 300 000 units of an antibiotic by IM injection. The label instructions state, "Add 5 mL of bacteriostatic water to yield 500 000 units per mL." Calculate the amount to give.

7. The order states ampicillin 1 g IV q6h. On hand is a vial of powdered medication. The label reads: 1 000 mg. If you add 1 mL of sterile water to the vial, calculate the amount you will administer.

8. A multiple-dose vial containing a powdered antibiotic is labeled Drug Q 10 g. The instructions state add 7.2 mL of sterile water to yield 10 mL total volume. What is the concentration in g per mL?

9. Refer to question 8 and calculate a dose of 1 500 mg.

10. Refer to question 8 and calculate a dose of 2.5 g.

Your Score: _____ /20 = _____ %

Exercise 6.6

Recognizing errors

For each of the following situations, indicate whether the calculation is correct. If incorrect, state the correct answer. (Value: 2 each)

1. The order is for 2 500 units SC bid and the available strength is 10 000 units/mL. Your co-worker has drawn up 2.5 mL. Is this correct?

2. The order is dimenhydrinate 50 mg IM stat. The available concentration is an ampule labeled 50 mg/mL. Is 1 ampule the correct amount to administer?

3. Fluphenazine decanoate 12.5 mg IM is ordered. The vial is labeled:
   10 mL of fluphenazine decanoate
   25 mg/mL
   Is the correct dosage 2 mL?

4. A co-worker asks you to double-check the drug dosage. The order is for 4 300 units, the label states 1 000 units/mL and the syringe indicates 4 mL has been drawn up. Correct?

5. An ampule is labeled 60 mg/2 mL. The order is for a stat dose of 45 mg. You calculate 1.5 mL. Validate. Correct?

Your Score: _____ /10 = _____ %

Exercise 6.7

Refer to the drug labels on page 104 and answer questions 1 through 15.

For each of the following drug orders state the correct amount to administer. Be sure to state the dosage strength of the drug, for example, give 1 mL of the 10 mg/mL strength. (Value: 2 each; 1 for calculation, 1 for validation)

1. Prostaphlin 500 mg IM q6h

2. Morphine 8 mg IM q3h

3. Morphine 7.5 mg SC q4h

4. Prostaphlin 125 mg IM q6h

5. Ampicillin 750 mg IM

(Q 6-15 Value: 1 each)

6. You have drawn up 0.6 mL of morphine sulfate 10 mg/mL solution. How many mg is contained in this volume?

Complete the box below for IM administration.

	Ancef	Prostaphlin	Polycillin-N
Volume of diluent	(7)	(8)	(9)
Resulting concentration of solution	(10)	(11)	(12)

13. Calculate 500 mg cefazolin sodium IM.

14. Calculate 300 mg oxacillin sodium IM.

15. You are to give 1.5 mL of reconstituted Polycillin-N. How many mg?

Your Score: _____ /20 = _____ %

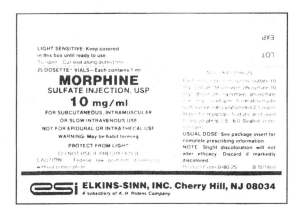

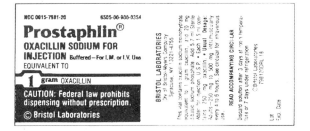

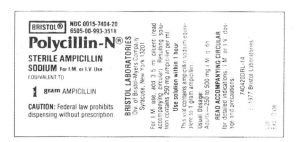

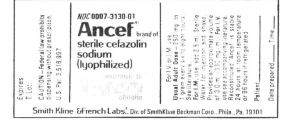

Additional Practice

Dosage calculation in the clinical setting requires several steps:

(1) Read the order

(2) Locate the medication (this varies considerably in settings)

(3) Read the label carefully (3 times)

(4) Calculate the dosage: Validate

(5) Administer the medication following the 5 rights.

This exercise is designed to provide further practice in
- reading labels
- calculating parenteral dosages
- reconstituting powders
- recognizing errors.

Refer to the Medication Cart on page 106. Read the order carefully. State the product you have chosen, e.g., Product B heparin 1 000 units/mL. Calculate and validate each medication order. (Value: 1 each)

PART A:

Order: morphine 8 mg IM stat
1. product
2. calculation
3. validation
4. shade in correct amount on syringe.

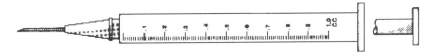

Order: cefazolin sodium 1 gram IM
concentration (approximately 330 mg/mL) – diluent plus powder = 3 mL or 1 g in 3 mL
5. product
6. amount of diluent
7. calculation
8. stability

Order: heparin 4 000 units SC
9. product
10. calculation
11. validation
12. shade in correct amount on syringe.

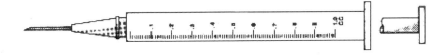

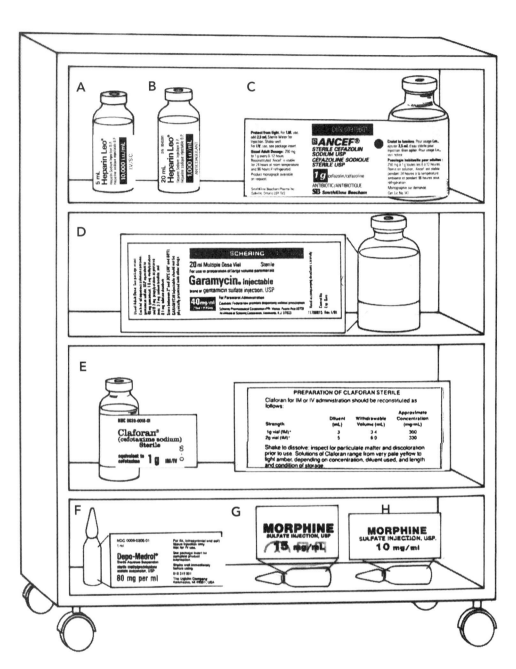

Medication Cart

Order: Depo-Medrol 60 mg IM
13. product
14. calculation
15. validation
16. instructions before using
17. what route is contraindicated?

Order: Claforan 500 mg IM
18. product
19. reconstitution
20. calculation
21. validation

Order: morphine 12 mg SC
22. product
23. calculation
24. validation
25. shade correct amount on syringes.

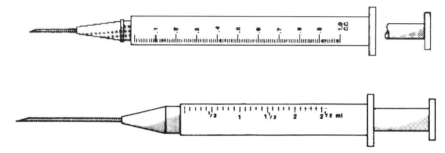

Order: gentamycin sulfate 50 mg IM
26. product
27. total volume in vial
28. concentration of solution
29. calculation
30. validation

Your Score: _____ **/30** = _____ %

PART B

Read the label. Answer questions 1-10. (Value: 1 each)

1. What diluent is recommended?

2. How long is reconstituted product stable at room temperature?

3. How long can this vial be stored in the refrigerator, after reconstitution?

4. What is the total weight of drug in the vial?

5. What is the generic name?

6. By what routes can drug be given?

7. Calculate 1 g dose.

8. Calculate 500 mg dose.

9. If 9.5 mL of diluent is added to vial and you have drawn up 2 mL, how much drug is contained in this volume?

10. If the order is for 750 mg, how many doses can be given from this vial?

Geopen®
carbenicillin disodium
Sterile
equivalent to
5 g of carbenicillin
For IM or IV use
CAUTION: Federal law prohibits
dispensing without prescription.

ROERIG ®
A division of Pfizer Inc. N.Y., N.Y. 10017

DIRECTIONS
IV Use:
Add 20 ml of Sterile Water for Injection.
After reconstitution dilute further to
desired volume with a suitable diluent.
IM Use:
Reconstitute with at least 7 ml of Sterile
Water for Injection. In order to facilitate
reconstitution, up to 17 ml of water for
injection may be used.

Amount of Diluent To Be Added To The 5 g Vial	Volume To Be Withdrawn For A 1 g Dose
7.0 ml	2.0 ml
9.5 ml	2.5 ml
12.0 ml	3.0 ml
17.0 ml	4.0 ml

For dosage information read
accompanying professional information.
After reconstitution, discard
any unused portion after 24 hours
(if stored at room temperature), or
after 72 hours (if refrigerated).
Store dry powder below 25°C.
MADE IN U.S.A. 3

Your Score: _____ /10 = _____ %

PART C

Refer again to the "Medication Cart" on page 106. Validate the following calculations. Is the answer correct? Is the answer expressed in the correct units? Is the choice of product correct? (Value: 2 each)

Order	Product	Dosage	Validation
1. heparin 3 000 units	heparin 1 000 units/mL	0.3 mL	
2. morphine 15 mg	morphine 10 mg/mL	1.5 mL	
3. Claforan 600 mg	Claforan 2 g	2 mL	
4. Depo-Medrol 40 mg	Depo-Medrol 80 mg/mL	0.5 mL	
5. Ancef 1 000 mg	Ancef 1 g	1 vial	

Your Score: _____ /10 = _____ %

Case Study

> Mrs. E.G., a 94-year-old woman is admitted to acute care for investigation of abdominal pain. No known allergies. Medication orders include:
> dimenhydrinate 50 mg IM q3–4h prn for nausea
> anileridine 15–25 mg IM q4–6h prn for pain
> acetaminophen liquid 325–650 mg PO q4h prn for pain
> cyanocobalamin injections of 100 mcg IM daily × 3 days

> Drug Supply:
>
> dimenhydrinate 1 mL ampule labeled 50 mg/mL
> anileridine 1 mL ampule labeled 25 mg/mL
> acetaminophen liquid, bottle labeled 160 mg/5 mL
> cyanocobalamin ampule labeled 100 mcg/mL

Administer minimum dose of anileridine IM stat.

1. Calculate
2. Validate

Administer dimenhydrinate IM stat.

3. Calculate
4. Validate

Administer today's dose of cyanocobalamin.

5. Calculate
6. Validate

Administer maximum dose of anileridine IM.

7. Calculate
8. Validate

Administer minimum dose of acetaminophen.

9. Calculate
10. Validate

Optional Activity

NOTE: Recall from module 4 that drug labels are not standardized. Reading labels requires attention and experience. You should always read the drug label 3 times: once as you take it from the shelf, drawer, or cupboard; again as you compare the label with the order; and again after you have calculated the dosage.

During a clinical experience, ask a nurse to show the variety of drug products and labels of powdered drug products. Select a few vials and/or boxes or package inserts and find the following:

- recommended diluent
- stability at room temperature and refrigerator
- total weight of drug in vial
- route of administration

Practice some calculations: look at the possible concentrations that can be prepared and calculate various doses.

POSTTEST

Instructions

Write the posttest without referring to any reference materials.

Correct the posttest using the answer guide. (Value: 1 each)

Be careful to include units with all answers (e.g., mg, mL, tab). Round decimal numbers to the nearest hundredth.

Read the label, answer questions 1-4

The label on the penicillin G potassium indicates that 9.6 mL of diluent was added at 1 300 hours on the seventeenth day of the month.

1. State the concentration of the solution.

2. Calculate 250 000 units IM stat.

3. State the hour and day of the month the drug is outdated.

4. Using another vial of penicillin G potassium, describe reconstitution and calculate 400 000 units IM.

    (a) reconstitution

    (b) calculation

    (c) validation

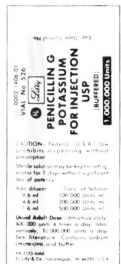

5. The order is perphenazine 3.5 mg IM stat. The ampule is labeled 5 mg/mL. Determine the correct volume to administer.

6. From hydrocortisone 100 mg/2 mL, determine the correct volume for 75 mg IM daily.

7. The order is: meperidine 75 mg IM prn. The ampule is labeled meperidine 100 mg/mL. Determine the correct volume to administer.

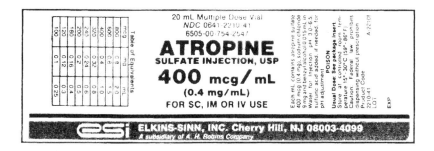

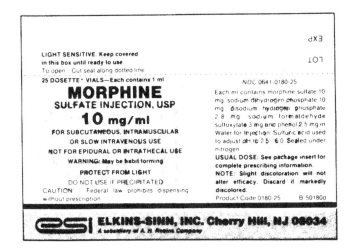

The order is morphine 8 mg IM and atropine sulfate 0.4 mg IM 1 hour preoperatively. Calculate:

8. The dosage of morphine

9. The dosage of atropine

10. The total volume in the syringe after the two drugs are drawn up. (These drugs can be mixed together for a short time.)

11. You have drawn up 0.6 mL of morphine. How many mg is contained in this volume?

12. Calculate: morphine 7.5 mg SC q3h prn

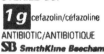

Protect from light. For I.M. use, add 2.5 mL Sterile Water for Injection. Shake well. For I.V. use, see package insert. **Usual Adult Dosage:** 250 mg to 1 g every 6-12 hours. Reconstituted 'Ancef' is stable for 24 hours at room temperature and 96 hours if refrigerated. Product monograph available on request.

SmithKline Beecham Pharma Inc. Oakville, Ontario L6H 5V2

DIN 01919601
ⓅANCEF®
STERILE CEFAZOLIN SODIUM USP
CÉFAZOLINE SODIQUE STERILE USP
1 g cefazolin/céfazoline
ANTIBIOTIC/ANTIBIOTIQUE
SB SmithKline Beecham

Craint la lumière. Pour usage i.m., ajouter 2.5 mL d'eau stérile pour injection. Bien agiter. Pour usage i.v., voir notice. **Posologie habituelle pour adultes :** 250 mg à 1 g toutes les 6 à 12 heures. Remis en solution, 'Ancef' est stable pendant 24 heures à la température ambiante et pendant 96 heures sous réfrigération. Monographie sur demande. Can. Lic. No. 147

173H951

Adult Dose Range: 1-12 grams daily in equally divided doses every 8-12 hours.
Reconstitution:
I.M.: Add 6 mL Sterile Water for Injection or Bacteriostatic Water for Injection; **shake well**; yields **270 mg** ceftizoxime/mL.
I.V.: Add 20 mL Sterile Water for Injection; **shake well**; yields **95 mg** ceftizoxime/mL.
I.V. Infusion: Reconstitute as above; further dilute with one of the recommended I.V. infusion solutions. Use reconstituted solution within 24 hours if kept at room temperature or 48 hours if refrigerated.
See Package Insert. Product Monograph available on request. Store powder at room temperature (15°C - 30°C).
under licence of Fujisawa Pharmaceutical Co., Ltd., Osaka, Japan
SmithKline Beecham Pharma Inc. Oakville, Ontario L6H 5V2

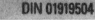

DIN 01919504
ⓅCEFIZOX®
STERILE CEFTIZOXIME SODIUM USP
CEFTIZOXIME SODIQUE STERILE USP
2 g ceftizoxime/vial/fiole
ANTIBIOTIC/ANTIBIOTIQUE
For Intramuscular or Intravenous Use
Pour usage intramusculaire ou intraveineux
SB SmithKline Beecham

Read the labels. Complete the box below.

	cefazolin sodium	ceftizoxime sodium
Shelf life after reconstitution	(13)	(14)
Route of administration	(15)	(16)
Total amount of drug in vial	(17)	(18)
Brand name	(19)	(20)

Your Score: _____ /20 = _____ %

100%   **Yes** — proceed to next module
       No — review and rewrite Posttest

Module 7: Intravenous Administration

Module Topics

- calculating rate of flow of intravenous infusions
- interpreting abbreviations related to intravenous therapy
- calculating fluid needs
- calculating kilojoules
- maintaining intravenous infusion (TKVO)
- continuous intravenous medication administration
- preparing and calculating IV medications for intermittent administration
- case studies

Calculating Rate of Flow of Intravenous Infusions

All intravenous fluids and medications must be administered precisely. The desired rate of flow must be calculated accurately and observed frequently during IV therapy.

The volume and type of IV fluid are ordered by the physician. The safe rate of intravenous administration is determined by many factors, including:

1. Age: infants and the elderly tolerate less fluid
2. Cardiovascular status
3. Site of infusion
4. Nature of the infusion; for example, irritating fluids or medications must be infused slowly to allow for adequate hemodilution

IV fluids are administered either by infusion pumps or by gravity drip. When a pump is used the rate of flow is expressed in mL per hour. For gravity drip, the rate must be calculated in drops per minute. This requires an additional step in the calculation. This module focuses on clinical situations involving gravity drip. Figure 7.1 illustrates IV administration sets.

To calculate the rate of flow for a gravity drip, you must know the following:

1. the volume of IV fluid ordered
2. the time for infusion
3. the drop factor; i.e., the calibration of the administration set in *drops per mL*

For example, macrodrop sets have a drop factor of 10, 15, or 20 drops per mL. In contrast, a minidrip produces a very small drop and 60 drops per mL (See Figure 7.1).

The physician's order for IV fluids is often written as "mL per hour." When using an infusion pump, simply set the pump at the ordered rate according to the manufacturer's instructions.

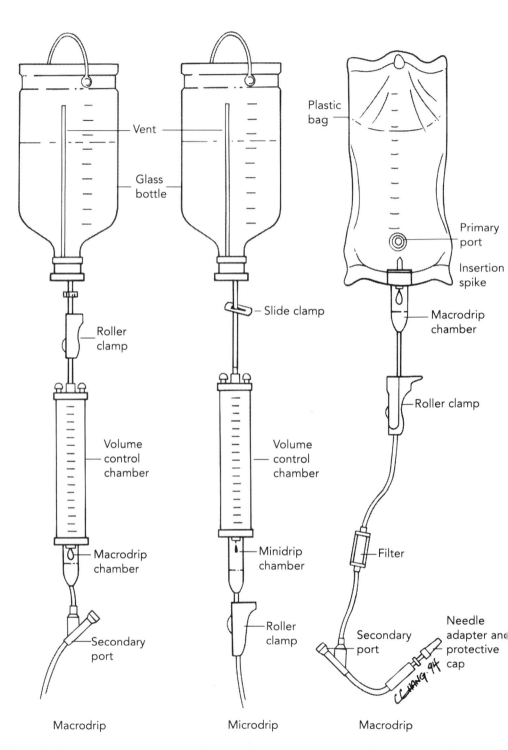

Figure 7.1 Intravenous administration sets from Clayton *Basic Pharmacology for Nurses*, 10/e, 1993.

For gravity drips, the rate can be converted to drops per minute, using a simple formula.

Formula

$$\frac{\text{volume of fluid (mL)}}{\text{time to infuse (minutes)}} \times \text{calibration of IV set} = \text{rate of flow (drops / minute)}$$

Example: Give 1 L over 10 hours.
Volume of fluid = 1 000 mL
Time to infuse = 10 h ´ 60 min = 600 minutes
Calibration of IV set (check IV tubing box).
For this problem use a minidrip set and 1 mL = 60 drops.

Use formula: $\dfrac{1\,000\,(\text{mL})}{600\,(\text{minutes})} \times 60\,(\text{drops / mL}) = \text{rate of flow} = 100\ \text{drops per minute}$

You may also use the formula to calculate the time required to infuse an IV solution. Alternatively, you can use ratio and proportion. Both methods are illustrated in the example.

Example:
The rate of flow of an IV is 100 drops/minute using a minidrip set (drop factor of 60 gtts/mL). How many hours are required to infuse one litre? Using the formula, insert all known values and use x for the unknown (time to infuse). Be sure to include all units to ensure an accurate problem statement.

$$\frac{1\,000\ \text{mL}}{\text{x minutes}} \times 60\,(\text{gtts / mL}) = 100\ \text{gtts / min}$$

$$\frac{60\,000}{\text{x}} = 100$$

x = 600 minutes (or 10 hours)

Ratio and Proportion
100 gtts/min = 100 mL/h (using the minidrip set)
100 mL:1 h = 1 000 mL:x h
x = 10 h

Before proceeding to the exercise, review the terms related to intravenous therapy in Table 7.1.

Primary

Secondary
or
Piggyback

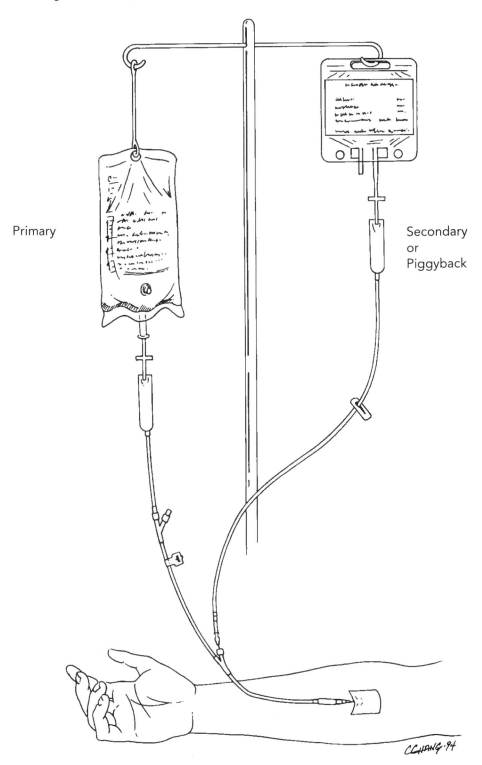

Fig. 7-2. Intravenous piggyback (IVPB) administration setup. Note that the smaller bottle is hung higher than the primary bottle. (Source: Gray: *Calculate with confidence*, 1994, p. 301)

Interpreting Abbreviations Related to Intravenous Therapy

Table 7.1: Terminology Related to IV Therapy

Term/Abbreviation	Definition
bolus	injection of medication over short period of time
D5W	solution of 5% dextrose in water
D5NS	solution of 5% dextrose in saline
NS	solution of normal (0.9%) saline
RL	Ringer's lactate
LVI	large volume infusion (e.g., 500–1000 mL)
SVI	small volume infusion (e.g., 25, 50, 100 mL minibag)
minidrip	also called microdrip: 60 drops/mL
macrodrip	also called regular drip: usually 10 drops/mL — check IV tubing set
primary line	see Figure 7.1
secondary line	see Figure 7.1
IVPB	intravenous piggyback (see Figure 7.2)
TKVO or TKO	slow rate of infusion "to keep vein open"
gtts	drops

Exercise 7.1

Complete the following exercise without referring to the previous text. Correct using the answer guide. State the rate of flow in whole numbers. (Value: 1 each)

1. Order #1: 1 L of normal saline over 8 hours. Calculate the rate of flow in drops per min using a minidrip with a drop factor of 60 drops/mL.

2. Order #2: 1 000 mL to run at 50 drops per minute. How many hours should this litre infuse using a minidrip (the drop factor is 60)?

Order #3: 3 000 mL of 5% dextrose over 24 hours.

3. For order #3, calculate the rate of flow, in drops per min using a regular set (the drop factor is 10).

4. For order #3, calculate the rate of flow, in drops per min using a minidrip set (the drop factor is 60).

5. The blood transfusion is infusing at 25 drops per minute, and the set is calibrated at 15 drops/mL. What is the hourly infusion rate, in mL?

Order #4: 3 000 mL in 24 hours.

6.   For order #4, calculate the total amount of fluid to infuse in 8 hours.

7.   For order #4, calculate the hourly infusion rate.

8.   For order #4, calculate the rate in drops per minute using a regular drip infusion set (the drop factor is 10).

9.   The ordered dose of a drug is dissolved in 100 mL to be infused over 1 hour. Calculate the rate of flow in drops per minute using a regular drip set (the drop factor is 10).

10. The order is to infuse 1 L of normal saline with an antineoplastic drug over 6 hours. Using a regular drip, with a drop factor of 15, calculate the rate of flow in drops per minute.

Your Score: _____ /10   =   _____ %

Exercise 7.2

This exercise provides additional practice calculating IV rate of flow. Check your responses with the answer guide. State rate of flow in whole numbers. (Value: 1 each)

Order 1: the patient is to receive 1 L of IV fluid in 8 hours.

1.   For order 1, calculate the number of mL per minute that the patient should receive.

2.   For order 1, calculate the rate of flow in drops per minute (the drop factor is 10).

7.   A 500 mL IV is infusing at the rate of 25 mL per hour. How many hours will it take for this IV to be infused?

Order 2: 1 L over 12 h.

3.   For order 2, calculate the volume to be infused in 1 hour.

4.   For order 2, calculate the rate of flow in drops per minute, using a minidrip set (the drop factor is 60).

8.   Ampicillin has been added to 50 mL of normal saline. The drug should be infused in 20 minutes. Calculate the rate of flow in gtts/min using a regular set with a drop factor of 1 mL = 10 drops.

Order 3: 2 L/day.

5.   For order 3, calculate the hourly rate of infusion.

6.   For order 3, calculate the rate in drops per minute (the drop factor is 15).

9.   The order is for 1 500 mL of saline over 24 hours. Calculate the infusion rate in gtts/min if the administration set delivers 20 drops/mL.

10. A litre of IV fluid has been running at 125 mL/hour for 3.5 hours. How much remains in the IV container?

11. The IV is ordered to run at 50 mL/hour. The administration set delivers 60 drops/mL. Calculate the infusion rate in drops per minute.

12. The IV container is labeled "infuse at 100 mL/hour." The administration set delivers 10 drops/mL. The IV is running at a rate of 20 drops per minute. Is this correct?

13. An IV container of 500 mL has infused for 1 hour at a rate of 100 mL/hour. A new rate of infusion is ordered at 50 mL/hour. Calculate the number of hours during which the remaining fluid will infuse.

14. The order is for 500 mL of blood over 3 hours. Calculate the rate of flow in gtts/min using a set with a drop factor of 15.

15. The IV is infusing at 125 drops per minute with a minidrip (the drop factor is 60). How long will it take to infuse 250 mL?

Your Score: _____ /15 = _____ %

Calculating Fluid Needs

Fluids may be ordered as L/day or mL/hour or according to body weight or surface area.
- One guide recommended for children is 1 500 mL/sq m/day.
- Another guide used for both children and adults is the following:

    100 mL/kg for the first 10 kg
    50 mL/kg for the next 10 kg
    20 mL/kg for all remaining kg

The following examples illustrate these concepts.

Example 1:

Calculate the hourly fluid replacement for a child with a body surface area of 0.6 sq meters.

1 500 mL per sq m = 1 500 × 0.6 = 900 mL
This child should receive 900 mL per day
or 900/24 = 37.5 (38) mL/hour.

Example 2:

Calculate the 24-hour fluid needs for an individual weighing 60 kg.

For the first 10 kg: 100 mL/kg = 1 000 mL
For the next 10 kg: 50 mL/kg = 500 mL
For the remaining 40 kg: 20 mL/kg = 800 mL
Total: 2 300 mL in 24 hours
or 2 300/24 = 95.8 (96) mL/hour.

Calculating Kilojoules

Sometimes you need to keep track of the kilojoules received in IV fluids. In a 5% dextrose solution, for example, every 100 mL of solution contains 5 g of dextrose. Each g of dextrose supplies 11.3 kilojoules (or 3.4 Kilocalories).

Exercise 7.3

Complete the exercise by using the guidelines above. Validate your responses, then correct using the answer guide. (Value: 3 each)

Calculate the daily fluid needs for each of the following individuals. An example is done for you.

1. A girl weighing 42 pounds
2. A child weighing 12 pounds, 4 oz
3. A woman weighing 50 kg
4. A teenager weighing 57 kg

Example: A man weighing 209 pounds

Convert 209 lbs to kg	= 95 kg
First 10 kg: 100 mL/kg	= 1 000 mL
Next 10 kg: 50 mL/kg	= 500 mL
Remaining 75 kg: 20 mL/kg	= 1 500 mL
TOTAL	3 000 mL/day

Calculate the total kilojoules supplied in a 24-hour period for each of the following individuals, assuming that 5% dextrose solution is used. Round your answer to the nearest whole number. An example is done for you.

5. A girl weighing 42 pounds
6. A child weighing 12 pounds, 4 oz
7. A woman weighing 50 kg
8. A teenager weighing 57 kg

Example: A man weighing 209 pounds requires 3 000 mL/day

3 000 mL contains x g dextrose
100 mL: 5 g = 3 000 mL: x g
$$x = 150 \text{ g}$$
Each g = 11.3 kj
150 g = 1 695 kj

Your Score: _____ /24 = _____ %

Maintaining Intravenous Infusions (TKVO)

In some situations, the physician wants to maintain the intravenous site but does not want to infuse significant amounts of fluid. This is referred to as "keeping the vein open" and may be abbreviated as TKO or TKVO. It is easier to maintain a very slow rate of infusion with a minidrip infusion set (60 gtts/mL) or with a pump.

Continuous Intravenous Medication Administration

Today many medications are given by the IV route which ensures complete absorption of the drug and rapid onset of action. Many institutions use an admixture program in which the drug in the IV solution is prepared and labelled by pharmacy and administered by the nurse. In others, the nurse must add the drug to the IV solution. This requires a knowledge of medications, mathematics, compatibility, and aseptic technique. Only the main points related to the skills of calculation will be addressed in this module.

CRITICAL POINT

It is essential to confirm the compatibility of the medication with the IV solution. Always check the package insert for specific instructions.

To deliver continuous IV medication, follow the instructions for preparing the IV solution and calculate the rate of flow. The following exercise provides practice with calculations related to this procedure using gravity drip. In some settings, it is policy to always use an infusion pump to deliver IV fluids with medications. Always check the policies in the clinical setting.

Exercise 7.4

Calculate all orders using a microdrip (60 gtts/mL). For each order, state the rate of flow of the IV solution and the amount of drug delivered per minute. (This is a useful practice in preparation for more complex situations which will be posed in the next modules.) An example is done for you. (Value: 2 each)

Order	Rate of flow (gtts/min)	Drug delivered/ minute
1000 mL with 20 mmol KCl over 8 h.	$\dfrac{1\,000\ mL}{8\ h \times 60\ min} \times 60\ gtts = rate$ 125 gtts/min	125 gtts/min = 2 mL (approx) $\dfrac{20\ mmol}{1\,000\ mL} = \dfrac{x\ mmol}{2\ mL}$ = 0.04 mmol KCL/min
1 000 mL with 40 mmol KCl over 10 h.	(1)	(2)
aminophylline 0.5 g in 500 mL and infuse over 10 h.	(3)	(4)

Read the following instructions adapted from a product monograph. Answer questions 5 to 10.

"For IV infusion: reconstitute with sterile water for injection. The reconstituted solution may be added to an appropriate IV bottle/bag containing any of the solutions listed. D5W; NS; lactated Ringer's; dextrose in saline." The instructions for the 1 gram and 2 gram vials appear in the table.

Vial size	Volume to be added to vial	Approximate available volume	Approximate concentration
1 g	9.5 mL	10 mL	100 mg/mL
2 g	19 mL	20 mL	100 mg/mL

Shake well until dissolved. Use within 24 h if kept at room temperature or 72 hours if stored under refrigeration.

Order: 1 g antibiotic in 1 L of NS over 12 h.

5. Which vial size should be used for the above order?

6. Describe reconstitution.

7. Describe preparation of IV solution.

8. Calculate rate of flow (minidrip) in drops per minute and mL/h.

9. How long can IV solution be used after preparation?

10. After only 3 hours, the IV must be discontinued. How much drug was received by the patient?

Your Score: _____ **/10** = _____ **%**

Preparing and Calculating Intravenous Medications for Intermittent Administration

In many situations, a medication is not given continuously. Instead, the drug is added to a small volume of fluid and infused over a short period of time.

Study Figure 7.1 and note that a drug could be added to the plastic bag, glass bottle, or the volume control chamber. Examine the figure and study the chamber. Note that any amount of fluid may be added from the primary bag by opening the clamp above the chamber. Medications may be added directly to the chamber via the port. For a small volume infusion (SVI) of very small volumes, using a chamber is ideal. It is always important to refer to medication literature to determine the recommended concentration strength. It will indicate how much fluid is required to dilute the drug sufficiently so that it will not harm the veins. It is also important to know the desired rate of administration.

> **CRITICAL POINT**
>
> IV administration is direct and not retrievable. Too rapid a rate can cause serious adverse effects. Always check the literature carefully or consult the pharmacy before preparing and administering a drug by the IV route.

For some situations, the medication is added to a second intravenous container, called a piggyback setup (IVPB) (Figure 7.2). This allows intermittent infusion of the medication over a short duration. The primary solution maintains the IV site or provides additional fluid. Study these sample problems and then complete the exercise for practice.

Example:

Order: methylprednisolone 80 mg in 50 mL NS and infuse over 30 minutes by IVPB.
Step 1: prepare medication. Drug is available in a 1 mL ampule, concentration of 80 mg/mL. Draw up 1 mL into a syringe and inject into a 50 mL minibag of NS through the rubber port.
Step 2: calculate rate of flow using a minidrip set.

$$\frac{\text{volume (mL)}}{\text{time (minutes)}} \times \text{calibration (gtts / mL)} = \frac{50}{30} \times 60 = 100 \text{ gtts / min}$$

Example:

Order: ampicillin 500 mg in 50 mL D5W and infuse over 20 minutes.
Step 1: prepare medication. Label of a 1 g vial of ampicillin states to add 3.5 mL sterile water to yield a solution of 250 mg/mL.
Known ratio: 250 mg/1 mL
Unknown ratio: 500 mg/x mL
Solve: 250 : 1 = 500 : x
   x = 2
Draw up 2 mL of drug solution and add to 50 mL minibag.
Step 2: calculate rate of flow using a minidrip set.

$$\frac{\text{volume (mL)}}{\text{time (minutes)}} \times \text{calibration (gtts / mL)} = \frac{50}{20} \times 60 = 150 \text{ gtts / min}$$

CRITICAL POINT

When reconstituting powdered medications, ensure that the drug is dissolved thoroughly. Shake well and allow to sit until any foam has settled. Examine for any precipitate or particulate matter; if this occurs, attempt to dissolve the drug or discard. If discolouration occurs, consult drug literature; if abnormal, discard.

CRITICAL POINT

IV bottles and bags are usually overfilled by 5% due to the manufacturing process and to ensure a minimum volume as stated on the product. For most clinical situations, especially when all of the solution (and therefore, all of the drug) will be infused, absolute accuracy with the volume is not required. Also, the volume may be increased slightly by adding the medication solution to the IV bottle/bag. In most cases, the overfill and the small volume of liquid medication added are not significant.

Now that you have learned how to prepare a medication for IV administration, review the steps. Cover the right column and answer the question posed in the left column then check your response.

Sequence of Questions	Responses
Step 1: What do you do first? What is the correct dosage? Order: ampicillin 500 mg in 25 mL minibag and infuse over 30 minutes. A 1 g vial of powder is reconstituted with 3.5 mL of sterile water, mixed thoroughly to produce a solution of 250 mg of ampicillin in each mL.	Determine the dosage to administer known ratio: 250 mg:1 mL unknown ratio: 500 mg:x mL proportion: 250:1 = 500:x $250x = 500$ $x = 2$ dose required = 2mL Validate using formula: $$\frac{\text{dose desired}}{\text{dose on hand}} \times \text{volume}$$ $$\frac{500}{250} \times 1 \text{ mL} = 2 \text{ mL}$$
Step 2: Prepare the IV solution.	Add 2 mL of the drug solution to a 25 mL minibag.
Step 3: Calculate the rate of flow in gtts/min using a minidrip set.	Use formula: $\dfrac{\text{volume}}{\text{time}} \times \text{calibration}$ $$\frac{25}{30} \times 60 = 50$$ Infuse at 50 drops/min
Challenge: the IV is infusing at 50 drops/minute. How much drug (ampicillin) is the patient receiving every minute?	Recall that the minibag has 500 mg drug dissolved in 25 mL solution. This means 500/25 = 20 mg per mL The IV set delivers 1 mL/60 drops; therefore 60:1 mL = 50:x mL $60x = 50$ $x = 50/60 = 0.83$ mL per minute Therefore, patient is receiving 20 mg : 1 mL = x drug mg : 0.83 mL $x = 20 \times 0.83$ $= 16.6$ mg per minute

Exercise 7.5

Complete the questions and correct using the answer guide. (Value: 1 each unless otherwise indicated).

For Orders #1-3, use a minidrip administration set (60 gtts/mL).

Order #1: amikacin 500 mg in 200 mL of NS infused over 1 hour.

1. Calculate flow rate in drops per minute.

2. How much of the drug (in mg) is delivered per minute?

Order #2: cefazolin sodium 250 mg IV q8h. Dilute in 50 mL of NS and infuse over 30 minutes.

3. Calculate flow rate in drops per minute.

4. How much of the drug (in mg) is delivered per minute?

Order #3: cephalothin sodium 2 g to be infused over 1 hour. Reconstitute the powdered drug and add to a 100 mL minibag of D5W.

5. Calculate flow rate in drops per minute for order #3.

6. Calculate the concentration of IV solution in mg/mL for ampicillin 500 mg in 50 mL minibag.

7. Penicillin 500 000 units is added to 100 mL and the rate of administration is ordered as 125mL/h. Calculate the time in minutes to infuse the drug. Calculate the concentration of the solution. (Value: 2)

Refer to the label and answer questions 8 and 9.

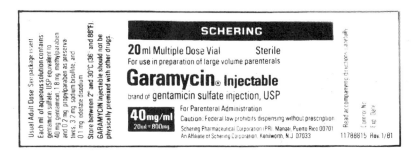

Order: gentamycin sulfate 80 mg IV q8h. The IV rate of flow is 50 mL/h. A 50 mL minibag and an infusion set (drop factor 20) are available.

8. Calculate the amount of drug to add to the minibag. Calculate the concentration of the solution (Value: 2)

9. Calculate the rate of flow in gtts/minute.

Read the package literature below and answer questions 10 through 15.

Product literature for cefazolin sodium (Ancef).

SINGLE DOSE VIAL RECONSTITUTION TABLE

Vial Size (mg)	Diluent	Volume to be added to Vial (mL)	Approximate Available Volume (mL)	Nominal Concentration (mg/mL)
500	Sodium Chloride Injection OR Sterile Water for Injection	2.0 3.8	2.2 4.0	225 125
1000	Sterile Water for Injection	2.5	3.0	334

For intermittent or Continuous Intravenous Infusion: Reconstitute as directed above. SHAKE WELL. Then further dilute reconstituted Ancef in 50 to 100 mL of Sterile Water for Injection or one of the Solutions for Intravenous Infusion.

Order: 250 mg Ancef IV q8h. The current IV is infusing at 100 mL/h.

10. Describe reconstitution of 0.5 g vial to yield solution of 125 mg/mL.

11. Calculate the amount of drug to add to 50 mL minibag. State the concentration of solution. (Value: 2)

12. Calculate the rate of flow using a microdrip set.

13. If the drug is started at 1300 hours, at what time will it be completely infused?

Order: 750 mg Ancef IV q8h. Infuse over 30 minutes.

14. Describe reconstitution of 1 g vial.

15. Calculate the amount of drug to add to 100 mL minibag.

16. Calculate rate of flow (set delivers 20 gtts/mL).

17. The IV is discontinued after 70 mL is absorbed. How much drug was received?

Your Score: _____ **/20** = _____ **%**

Exercise 7.6

Complete this exercise for further practice preparing IV medication solutions. Express rate of flow in whole numbers.

The following reconstitution device is to be used for order #1.

Reconstitution device: the minibag is squeezed which forces fluid into the vial. Mix powder thoroughly then invert with vial on top and squeeze minibag until fluid from vial flows into bag. This device provides the advantages of immediate reconstitution without adding an additional volume of liquid to the minibag and also reduces risks of contamination during the process of medication preparation.

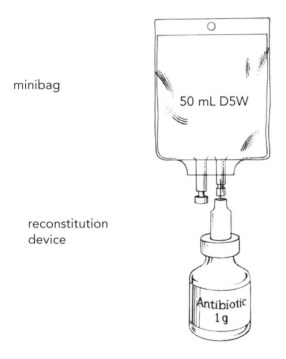

minibag

50 mL D5W

reconstitution device

Antibiotic 1 g

Order #1: Antibiotic 1 g IV q8h. IV rate is 100 mL/h. Add drug to 50 mL minibag.

1. Calculate strength of IV solution produced (mg/mL).

2. Calculate infusion time in minutes.

3. Calculate rate of flow in gtts/min using a set that delivers 20 gtts/mL.

Read the label and order #2 to answer questions 4 through 8.

Order #2: Ampicillin sodium 1 g IV.

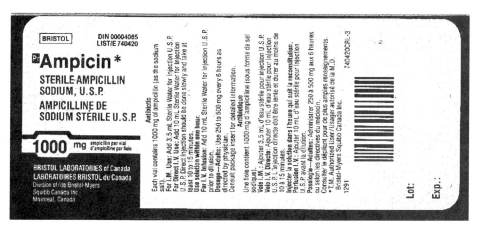

4. Describe reconstitution for IV use.

5. Package insert indicates that IV solution must not exceed concentration of 30 mg/mL. Which size minibag can be used: 25 mL? 50 mL?

6. Calculate rate of flow to infuse in 30 minutes by gravity drip with a drop factor of 10.

7. In some clinical settings, the drug may be given by direct IV injection. What period of time is recommended for direct IV administration of this drug?

8. The IV was initiated at 0800 h and interrupted at 0820 h. Assuming the rate of flow was consistent, how much drug would have been delivered during that time?

9. An IVPB with 500 mg of drug in 50 mL of solution is infusing at 100 mL/h. How much drug is infused in 15 minutes?

10. For #9, how much fluid is infused in 20 minutes?

Your Score: _____ **/10** = _____ **%**

Additional Practice

Further practice with IV rates and medication administration is offered in this exercise. Answer questions and correct using the Answer Guide. (Value: 1 for each calculation).

1. Calculate the rate of flow in drops/min for this order: 500 mL over 3 hours. The drop factor is 10.

2. Using an administration set with a drop factor of 15 and an infusion rate of 15 gtts/min, how much time would be required to infuse 60 mL?

3. A 100 mL minibag infusion at 50 gtts/min (the drop factor is 60) is initiated at 1130 hours. At what time should it be completely infused?

4. An IV is infusing at 125 mL/h. How many mL will be absorbed in a 12-hour shift?

5. An IV infuses at 20 gtts/min (drop factor is 10) for 4 hours. How much fluid has infused?

Order #1: cephalothin sodium loading dose of 2 g IV before surgery. On hand is a vial labelled 1 g of cephalothin sodium with 63 mg of sodium per gram. The instructions are to dilute the drug with 20 mL of sterile water for injection and add to the IV solution. The IV of NS is infusing at 100 mL/hour. Calculate the answers to questions 6-9.

6. Describe the reconstitution of the required amount of drug to provide the loading dose.

7. State the rate of flow of the IV if the infusion set delivers 10 gtts/mL.

8. State the amount of sodium the patient will receive from the drug with this loading dose.

9. Maintain the original rate of flow of the IV infusion and state the volume of IV fluid to add the cephalothin sodium dose and infuse over 1 hour.

Order #2: 250 mg IV over 30 minutes. The minibag is labelled 250 mg/100 mL. The drop factor is 10 drops/mL.

10. Calculate the rate of flow in drops per minute.

11. State the concentration of the minibag solution.

Order #3: ampicillin 500 mg IV q4h. An admixture solution of ampicillin 500 mg in a 50 mL minibag is available. The infusion drop factor is 60 gtts/mL. The drug should infuse over 30 minutes and the primary IV is running at 125 mL/hour. Calculate the answers to questions 12-15.

12. State the rate of flow in gtts/min for the primary IV.

13. State the rate of flow to infuse the drug.

14. What is the total amount of ampicillin the patient will receive in 24 hours?

15. Calculate the total volume of fluid infused in 24 hours, including the minibags and the primary IV solution. (Recall that the primary infusion is stopped while the minibag with the medication is running.)

Your Score: **/15**   =   **%**

Case Studies

This exercise will illustrate calculations when several IV solutions and medications are ordered for one patient.

Case Study 1

Mrs. A.J., a 49-year-old patient, has an intravenous infusion of D5W running at 100 mL/hour. She is also receiving:
cefotetan 1.5 g q12h delivered in a 50 mL minibag of D5W over 30 min at 0600 and 1800 h.
methylprednisolone 80 mg q8h in a 50 mL minibag of NS over 30 minutes at 0800, 1600, and 2400 h.

Answer questions 1-5 for Case Study 1.

1. Total NS delivered in 24 hours.

2. Total D5W delivered in 24 hours.

3. The IV has infused from 0600 to 1900 h. How much NS and D5W have been absorbed?

4. For the same time period, calculate the total amount of each drug:

   (a) cefotetan

   (b) methylprednisolone

5. Using a minidrip infusion set, calculate the rate of flow in drops per minute for each IV:

   (a) primary solution

   (b) cefotetan

   (c) methylprednisolone

> ### Case Study 2
>
> Miss Brown has an IV of NS infusing at 125 mL/h which often slows down due to her positioning and movement. The physician states that the IV fluid rate must be maintained or increased to ensure adequate fluid intake. Calculate all adjustments in rate that must be made to accomplish this goal. The #1 IV of NS, a 1 000 mL bag, is commenced at 0800 h.

Complete the table for Case Study 2.

Time	IV	Amount remaining	Amount absorbed	Rate Adjusted rate
0800	#1 NS	1000	0	125 mL/h
0900	#1 NS	900	100	(1)
1000	#1 NS	750	250	125 mL/h
1100	#1 NS	600	400	(2)
1200	#1 NS	450	550	(3)

POSTTEST

Instructions

Write the posttest without referring to any reference materials.

Correct the posttest using the answer guide.

Be careful to:

a. *Include the appropriate units of measure with the answer when necessary*

b. *Round decimal numbers to the nearest whole number*

c. *Write decimal numbers correctly, using a zero to the left of the decimal point when necessary*

(Value: 3 each 1 for calculation, 1 for validation, 1 for including correct units and rounding)

You should deduct marks if your answers are not expressed correctly, as indicated above.

If your score is 100 percent, congratulations! You are ready for the "real world" of calculating most medications for administration to patients in the clinical setting — assuming, of course, that you have mastered the preceding modules. Module 8 offers more practice if you need it. Module 9 explains more complex but less common clinical calculations. You will want to complete Module 9 before practicing in the following settings: pediatrics, coronary or critical care units, emergency, and neonatal units.

If you don't achieve 100 percent, review the learning package in this module and rewrite the posttest.

For each of the following clinical situations, calculate as directed:

Order 1: 1 000 mL q8h.

1. For order 1, calculate the rate of flow in drops/min using a minidrip with a drop factor of 60.

2. For order 1, calculate the rate of flow in drops/min using a set with a drop factor of 10.

Order 2: aminophylline 50 mg per hour, to be given by continuous infusion. The intravenous manual instructions are as follows: "dilute to a concentration of 1 mg/ mL of dextrose or normal saline."

3. For order 2, calculate the volume of fluid required for a 2-hour infusion.

4. For order 2, calculate the rate of flow in drops/min using a minidrip set (the drop factor is 60).

5. For order 2, a 50 mL minibag is marked in this way: "contains 50 mg of aminophylline." It is infusing at 50 drops per minute (the drop factor is 60). How much of the drug is infused in 30 minutes?

6. For order 2, calculate the length of time to infuse this drug if 500 mg is added to 500 mL and a minidrip set is used (the drop factor is 60).

Order 3: 250 mg q6h. The patient has an IV infusion with a minidrip set (the drop factor is 60). The intravenous manual instructions are: "dilute to 5 mg/mL and infuse over 30 minutes."

7. For order 3, calculate the volume of fluid required to dilute the drug.

8. For order 3, calculate the rate of flow in drops/min.

Order 4: 1 000 mL q8h x 24 hours. After 3 hours, with a regular set (the drop factor is 10), only 300 mL are absorbed.

9. For order 4, calculate the volume that should have infused in the 3-hour period.

10. For order 4, calculate the new rate of flow in drops/min for the remaining 700 mL to be absorbed within the ordered time period.

Your Score: /30 =   %

Module 8: Clinical Challenges and Case Studies

Module Topics

- insulin preparations
- mixing insulins
- protocol for IV heparin
- case studies

Introduction

This module provides an opportunity to learn the skills involved for more complex calculation, including the technique of mixing two medications in the same syringe. A trend in medication administration is the use of protocols to guide calculation and titration of frequently-changing doses. A sample protocol for heparin administration will provide the example for this skill. This module also provides clinical simulation of dosage calculations through case studies.

Insulin preparations

Insulin is a hormone, produced by the pancreas, that can be administered SC for the treatment of diabetes mellitus. It can be obtained from animal sources or made synthetically. It is discussed in this book because of the challenges of total accuracy and the technique of mixing two insulin preparations in the same syringe.

In the past, insulin was produced only from beef and pork pancreatic sources. Today, human insulin is prepared biosynthetically, using recombinant DNA technology, or semisynthetically, using enzymatic modification technology. Like all hormones, insulin is required in small amounts; for example, the human body makes about 25 units daily.

Insulin preparations are categorized by their onset and duration of action.

A. Rapid action

Regular crystalline zinc insulin or (CZI) is clear, rapid acting and of short duration. The label may indicate regular with the name Toronto or with an R.

B. Modified insulins

These are made with large protein molecules of protamine and are cloudy white suspensions with a slower onset and longer duration of action. Note that these suspensions must be gently rotated before administration to ensure a homogeneous mixture. The label may indicate N or NPH (neutral pH) or the word isophane.

C. Lente insulins

The lente insulins are formulated with zinc into large crystals that delay absorption and onset of action. Semilente is turbid, has a rapid onset, but a slightly longer duration than regular insulin. Lente is intermediate acting, whereas ultralente is the longest acting insulin.

D. Mixed Preparations

For convenience, some insulins are a mixture of regular and modified preparations in one vial. For example, Humulin 30/70 has 30% regular human insulin injection with 70% intermediate-acting (isophane) insulin. An injection of 1 mL of this suspension would provide 30 units of regular and 70 units of modified insulin.

CRITICAL POINT

All insulin preparations are provided in multidose vials in the concentration strength of 100 units/mL. This is an important safety precaution to assist with accurate dosage calculations. Always read the order and label carefully. There are many different insulin preparations and an error could be very serious.

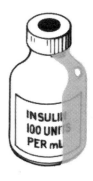

Most patients receive insulin in small doses; e.g., 5 units. This requires a very careful technique and accurate equipment. Insulin syringes are supplied in 0.3 mL (or 30 units), 0.5 mL (or 50 units) and 1 mL (or 100 units) sizes. The syringe is designed with the needle attached and, therefore, there is no "dead space volume;" the hub of many needles contains as much as 0.1 mL, equal to 10 units of insulin — a significant amount.

Compare the two syringes in Figure 8.1.

Regular syringe showing
dead space volume (DSV)

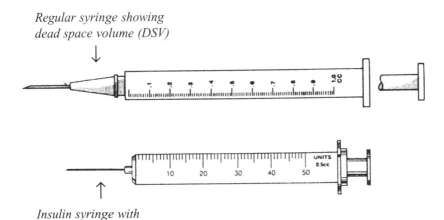

Insulin syringe with
no DSV

Exercise 8.1

Study the insulin labels on page 137 carefully to become acquainted with the variety of types of insulins. Complete the table. An example is done for you.

Product/name	Type
A. Novolin ge Toronto	rapid acting
B. (1)	(2)
C. (3)	(4)
D. (5)	(6)

Study the premixed insulin labels on page 138 and complete the table.

Product	Units/mL regular insulin	Units/mL modified insulin
A.	20 units/mL	80 units/mL
B.	(7)	(8)
C.	(9)	(10)
D.	(11)	(12)
E.	(13)	(14)

Calculate the amounts of regular and modified insulin in each of the following volumes of premixed insulins.

15.   14 units of Humulin 50/50: _____ units of regular and _____ units modified insulin.

16.   50 units of Humulin 20/80: _____ units of regular and _____ units modified insulin.

17.   30 units of Humulin 30/70: _____ units of regular and _____ units modified insulin.

18.   70 units of Humulin 50/50: _____ units of regular and _____ units modified insulin.

19.   40 units of Humulin 10/90: _____ units of regular and _____ units modified insulin.

20.   25 units of Humulin 20/80: _____ units of regular and _____ units modified insulin.

Your Score: _____ /20 = _____ %

Insulin Labels

A.

SAMPLE LABEL

Connaught
Novo Nordisk

10 ml   100 units per ml/unités par ml

Novolin®ge Toronto

Insulin Injection,
Human Biosynthetic
(Regular)

Insuline humaine
biosynthétique, injectable
(Régulière)

HUMAN/HUMAINE   DIN 02024233

B.

Connaught
Novo Nordisk

10 ml   100 units per ml/unités par ml

Novolin®ge NPH

Insulin Isophane,
Human Biosynthetic

Insuline humaine
biosynthétique, isophane

HUMAN/HUMAINE   DIN 02024225

C.

SAMPLE LABEL

Connaught
Novo Nordisk

10 ml   100 units per ml/unités par ml

Novolin®ge Lente

Insulin Zinc Suspension - Medium,
Human Biosynthetic

Insuline zinc humaine
biosynthétique, à action
intermédiaire, en suspension

HUMAN/HUMAINE   DIN 02024241

D.

Lilly   **DIN 00587737**

HI-310   10 mL

U-100   **100 Units • unités/mL**

Humulin **N**

NPH insulin isophane,
human biosynthetic
(r DNA origin)
NPH insuline humaine
biosynthétique (source ADN r)
isophane

E.

Lilly   **DIN 00586714**

HI-210   10 mL

U-100   **100 Units • unités/mL**

Humulin **R**

REGULAR insulin injection,
human biosynthetic
(r DNA origin)
RÉGULIÈRE insuline humaine
biosynthétique (source ADN r)
injectable

Premixed Insulin Labels

A.

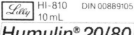

HI-810 DIN 00889105
10 mL

Humulin® 20/80

20% insulin injection
80% insulin isophane
human biosynthetic (r DNA Origin)
100 Units per mL

insulines humaines biosynthétiques
injectable 20% et isophane 80%
(source ADN r)
100 unités par mL

Lot.
Exp.

See insert for directions
Voir le mode d'emploi dans le
dépliant de conditionnement
U-100
SHAKE CAREFULLY
AGITER AVEC SOIN

LILLY FRANCE S.A., F-67640
FEGERSHEIM, FRANCE
YC 2090 GECAX

B.
HI-710 DIN 00795879
10 mL

Humulin® 30/70

30% insulin injection
70% insulin isophane
human biosynthetic (r DNA Origin)
100 Units per mL

insulines humaines biosynthétiques
injectable 30% et isophane 70%
(source ADN r)
100 unités par mL

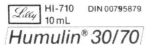

Lot.
Exp.

See insert for directions
Voir le mode d'emploi dans le
dépliant de conditionnement
U-100
SHAKE CAREFULLY
AGITER AVEC SOIN

LILLY FRANCE S.A., F-67640
FEGERSHEIM, FRANCE
YC 0604 GECAX

C.
HI-1510 DIN 00889121
10 mL

Humulin® 50/50

50% insulin injection
50% insulin isophane
human biosynthetic (r DNA Origin)
100 Units per mL

insulines humaines biosynthétiques
injectable 50% et isophane 50%
(source ADN r)
100 unités par mL

Lot.
Exp.

See insert for directions
Voir le mode d'emploi dans le
dépliant de conditionnement
U-100
SHAKE CAREFULLY
AGITER AVEC SOIN

LILLY FRANCE S.A., F-67640
FEGERSHEIM, FRANCE
YC 2650 GECAX

D.
HI-910 DIN 00889113
10 mL

Humulin® 10/90

10% insulin injection
90% insulin isophane
human biosynthetic (r DNA Origin)
100 Units per mL

insulines humaines biosynthétiques
injectable 10% et isophane 90%
(source ADN r)
100 unités par mL

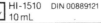

Lot.
Exp.

See insert for directions
Voir le mode d'emploi dans le
dépliant de conditionnement
U-100
SHAKE CAREFULLY
AGITER AVEC SOIN

LILLY FRANCE S.A., F-67640
FEGERSHEIM, FRANCE
YC 2100 GECAX

E.
HI-1610 DIN 00889091
10 mL

Humulin® 40/60

40% insulin injection
60% insulin isophane
human biosynthetic (r DNA Origin)
100 Units per mL

insulines humaines biosynthétiques
injectable 40% et isophane 60%
(source ADN r)
100 unités par mL

Lot.
Exp.

See insert for directions.
Voir le mode d'emploi dans le
dépliant de conditionnement.
U-100
SHAKE CAREFULLY
AGITER AVEC SOIN

LILLY FRANCE S.A., F-67640
FEGERSHEIM, FRANCE
YC 2110 GECAX

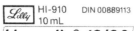

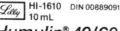

Mixing Insulins

Some medications may be drawn up together in one syringe for injection. One example is mixing morphine with atropine in a single syringe for IM injection before surgery. Often regular insulin (rapid acting, clear form) is mixed with a modified insulin (an opaque white suspension).

Principles to follow for mixing two insulins include:

1.   use the standard procedure for preparing any injection
     - aseptic technique
     - read medication order
     - read label three times

2.   use technique to avoid contaminating one insulin with the other. Figure 8.2 illustrates the steps for mixing two insulins. The following example reviews the steps.

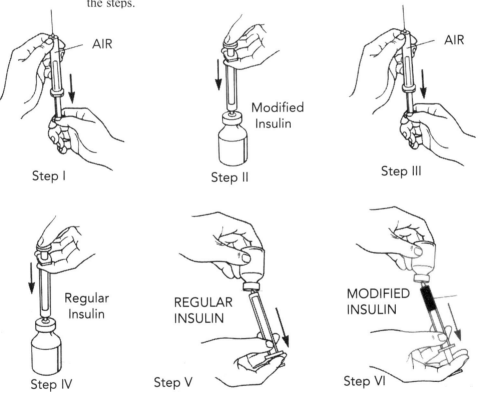

Step I   —   AIR

Step II   —   Modified Insulin

Step III   —   AIR

Step IV   —   Regular Insulin

Step V   —   REGULAR INSULIN

Step VI   —   MODIFIED INSULIN

CRITICAL POINT

When mixing insulins, only those from the same source can be mixed: e.g., pork and pork; human and human.

Many agencies have a policy whereby the procedure of mixing insulins must be verified by two nurses. Check each specific clinical setting for policies regulating medication administration.

Procedure for mixing two insulins:

1.   add the two amounts to determine the final volume.

2.   select an appropriate syringe size.

3.   create a positive pressure in both vials by injecting a volume of air equal to the required volume of liquid to be withdrawn. Begin with the modified insulin vial.

4.   withdraw the required amount of regular insulin.

5.   withdraw the required amount of NPH insulin.

Example

1) Give regular insulin 8 units and NPH 14 units.
   8 units and 14 units = 22 units

2) A 30-units (or 0.3 mL) syringe is best.

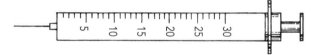

3) Rotate NPH vial gently to mix suspension.
   Inject the equivalent of 14 units of air into NPH vial.
   Inject the equivalent of 8 units of air into regular insulin vial.

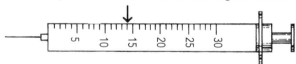

4) Withdraw 8 units of regular insulin.

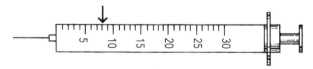

5) Insert needle into NPH insulin being very careful not to push on plunger (not to lose any of the dose of regular insulin). Withdraw required amount of NPH by pulling plunger to 22 units.

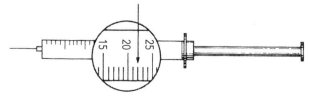

Exercise 8.2

Practice the steps of mixing two insulins. Verify the responses with the Answer Guide.

Refer to the labels on pages 137 and 138.

1. Order: regular insulin 10 units and NPH 18 units.
   State which products you are using: (1) _____ and (2) _____
   Calculate total volume:
   Procedure: rotate suspension to ensure homogeneous mixture: inject equivalent of
   (3) ___ units of air into (4) _____ vial; inject equivalent of (5) _____ units of air
   into (6) _____ vial; withdraw (7) _____ units of (8) _____ insulin and
   (9) _____ units of (10) _____ insulin (for a total of (11) _____ units).

2. Order: Toronto insulin 14 units and NPH 26 units.
   State which products you are using: (12) _____ and (13) _____
   Calculate total volume:
   Procedure: rotate suspension to ensure homogeneous mixture: inject equivalent of
   (14)___units of air into (15)_____vial; inject equivalent of (16)_____ units of
   air into (17) _____ vial; withdraw (18) _____ units of (19) _____
   insulin and (20) _____ units of (21) _____ insulin (for a total of (22) ____ units).

3. Order: Humulin R insulin 10 units and Humulin N 20 units.
   State which products you are using: (23) _____ and (24)_____
   Calculate total volume:
   Procedure: rotate suspension to ensure homogeneous mixture: inject equivalent of
   (25)___units of air into (26) _____vial; inject equivalent of (27)_____units of
   air into (28) _____ vial; withdraw (29) _____ units of (30) _____
   insulin and (31) _____ units of (32) _____ insulin (for a total of (33) ___ units).

4. Order: Humulin R insulin 7 units and Humulin N 11 units.
   State which products you are using: (34) _____ and (35) _____
   Calculate total volume:
   Procedure: rotate suspension to ensure homogeneous mixture: inject equivalent of
   (36)___units of air into (37)_____vial; inject equivalent of (38)_____units of
   air into (39) _____ vial; withdraw (40) _____ units of (41) _____
   insulin and (42) _____ units of (43) _____ insulin (for a total of (44) ___ units).

Your Score: _____ /44 = _____ %

Calculating Intravenous Heparin by Protocol

The anticoagulant, heparin, is administered by the SC and the IV routes. The dosage is frequently adjusted depending on the individual's response to the drug. Laboratory monitoring of the aPTT is required to adjust heparin doses. Many clinical settings have adopted a protocol to provide guidelines for heparin therapy. Review the protocol for heparin therapy and study the example, then proceed to the exercise.

Protocol for Intravenous Heparin Therapy

Initiate therapy with a bolus/loading dose of 5 000 units IV, then use a standard heparin infusion of 25 000 units in 500 mL of D5W. Run IV at prescribed rate using an infusion pump. (See table)

Monitor aPTT and adjust the infusion rate according to the laboratory value.

aPTT in seconds	Stop infusion for..	Rate change	Repeat aPTT
< 45	0 minutes	+ 6 mL/h	4–6 hours
46–54	0 minutes	+ 3 mL/h	4–6 hours
55–85	0 minutes	0	in am
86–110	30 minutes	– 3 mL/h	4–6 hours after restarting heparin
> 110	60 minutes	– 6 mL/h	4–6 hours after restarting heparin

Example: You have an IV infusion premixed with heparin 25 000 units/500 mL bag of D5W. This is equivalent to 50 units/mL. You are instructed to commence IV at 32 mL/h. This means that the patient is receiving (32 x 50) 1 600 units of heparin per hour. The aPTT is done and the laboratory telephones the results. The patient's aPTT is 48 seconds. Find this value on the chart (46-54) and read that you will not stop the IV infusion, but will increase the rate of flow by 3 mL/hour. Now the patient is receiving an additional 150 units of heparin per hour (3 × 50 = 150). The new rate is (32 + 3) 35 mL/h, and the patient is now receiving 1 600 + 150 = 1 750 units/h. Four hours later, the aPTT is repeated and the new value is 90 seconds. Using the protocol, you would stop the infusion for 30 minutes and resume at a new rate by decreasing by 3 mL/h. (NOTE that the patient is now receiving the original rate.) You would order another aPTT in 4-6 hours after you have restarted the infusion.

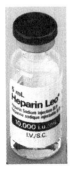
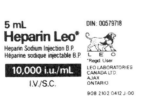

5 mL   DIN: 00579718
Heparin Leo*
Heparin Sodium Injection B.P.
Héparine sodique injectable B.P.   L E O
*Regd. User
10,000 i.u./mL   LEO LABORATORIES
CANADA LTD
AJAX
I.V./S.C.   ONTARIO
9OB 2102 0412 J·00

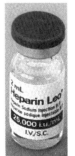
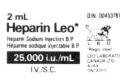

2 mL   DIN: 00453781
Heparin Leo*
Heparin Sodium Injection B.P.
Héparine sodique injectable B.P.   L E O
*Regd. User
25,000 i.u./mL   LEO LABORATORIES
CANADA LTD
AJAX
I.V./S.C.   ONTARIO

Exercise 8.3

Review the protocol for heparin therapy and read the Case Study. Answer the questions carefully and verify with the Answer Guide. If you have problems at any stage of the exercise, check with the Answer Guide before proceeding, or review the example. (Value: 1 each) Refer to the labels on page 142.

Case Study

Mrs. J.R. is being treated for thrombophlebitis. The order is "Administer a bolus of 5 000 units IV over 15 minutes at 0900 h. Commence IV heparin infusion at 20 units/kg/hour at 0915 h. Mrs. J.R. weighs 110 pounds. Four hours later (1315 h) the aPTT is 40 seconds and the rate is adjusted. Six hours later (1915 h) the aPTT is 52 seconds and the rate is adjusted. Four hours later (2315 h) the aPTT is 60 seconds. The IV infusion continues and the aPTT is drawn in the am. At 0945 h the lab calls with a new aPTT of 88 seconds. IV infusion is stopped for 30 minutes and the new rate is set at 1015 h.

---

1. Calculate the bolus infusion. State which product to use.

2. Validate the bolus injection. (NOTE: some agencies require verification of an IV medication by another professional.)

3. Describe the preparation of the IV infusion. State which product to use.

    (NOTE: some agencies have admixture programs in which IV infusions are premixed by the pharmacy. However, even with these programs, nurses may have to mix the medication.)

4. Calculate the initial rate of flow for the IV at 0915 h.

5. Calculate the adjusted rate of flow for the infusion at 1315 h.

6. State the number of units/hour Mrs. R. is receiving at the new rate.

7. Calculate the adjusted rate of flow for the IV infusion at 1915 h.

8. State the number of units/hour Mrs. R. is receiving at the new rate.

9. Calculate the total IV fluid intake from 0915 h to 2315 h.

10. Calculate the total heparin dosage received over 24 hour period (including the bolus) beginning at 0900 h – 0915 h the following am.

Your Score: _____ /10   =   _____ %

Case Studies

CRITICAL POINT

This situation is presented to illustrate the types of inconsistencies that occur in the clinical setting. Drugs may be ordered by generic or trade names. Medication cupboards may be stocked by generic or trade names, and a specific drug may be available in a variety of strengths.

Read Case Study #1. Locate the medication in the "Medication Cupboard" below. Calculate the amount to give for each medication as indicated. Use this schedule for administration times.

daily: 0800h
bid: 0800h and 2000h
tid: 0800h, 1600h and 2200h
q12h: 0800h and 2000h

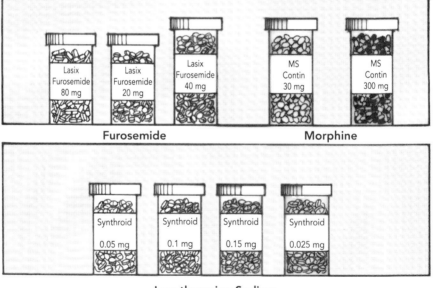

Case Study 1

Orders for Miss XR are:
Lasix 80 mg PO (even days)
Lasix 60 mg PO (odd days)
morphine sustained release 300 mg PO q12h and 30 mg prn for breakthrough pain
levothyroxine sodium 0.1 mg daily
Ativan 1 mg PO bid prn

A. Calculations for Miss XR for 0800h for 01-01-95.

Drug ordered	Dose	Product used and amount administered
Lasix	(1)	(2)
morphine	(3)	(4)
levothyroxine sodium	(5)	(6)

B. Additional questions.

7. What is the total daily dose of morphine, assuming there is no breakthrough pain?

8. If Miss XR experiences breakthrough pain, what would you do given the medication supply on hand?

9. When making the bed, you find a small flat yellow pill. How could you identify this pill?

10. On the 31st day of the month, Miss XR received one tablet of furosemide 80-mg strength. Did she receive the correct dose?

Case Study 2

Mr. J.A., an 81-year-old retired farmer is admitted for investigation of chest pain, shortness of breath, and weight loss. He has a history of asthma.
Present medications include:
Procan SR 0.75 g PO q6h
Cardizem 60 mg PO qid ac and hs
Nitro Patch: Nitro-Dur, 0.2 mg/h, apply 0800 h and remove 2200 h
Lasix 40 mg PO q am
nitroglycerin SL tab 0.3 mg at bedside.

Refer to drug labels below.

Calculate all doses for 0800 h administration for Mr. J.A. Use this schedule:

q am: 0800 h

qid ac and hs: 0800 h, 1200 h, 1600 h, and 2200 h

q6h: 0600 h, 1200 h, 1800 h, and 2200 h

Be sure to specify which product you are using from the labels illustrated below.

Drug name	Dose ordered	Product used	Amount given
(1)	(2)	(3)	(4)
(5)	(6)	(7)	(8)
(9)	(10)	(11)	(12)

(A)

procainamide HCL
Procan SR
750 mg tablets

(B)

diltiazem HCL
Cardizem
30 mg tablets

(C)

furosemide
Lasix
80 mg tablets

(D)

nitroglycerin SL
0.3 mg tablets

(E)

procainamide HCL
Procan SR
500 mg tablets

(F)

diltiazem HCL
Cardizem
60 mg tablets

(G)

diltiazem HCL SR
60 mg tablets
Cardizem SR

(H)

furosemide
Lasix
40 mg tablets

(I)

Nitro-Dur
0.2 mg/h

Case Study 3

Refer to the product information on Cefizox and the drug label for Colace to answer the questions on the following page.

RECONSTITUTION

STANDARD VIALS (1 GRAM AND 2 GRAMS)

For Intramuscular Injection: Reconstitute with Sterile Water for Injection or Bacteriostatic Water for Injection.

Reconstitution Table for Standard Vials – I.M. Injection			
Vial Size	Diluent to be Added to Vial	Approximate Available Volume	Approximate Average Concentration
1 g	3.0 mL	3.7 mL	270 mg/mL
2 g	6.0 mL	7.4 mL	270 mg/mL

Shake well until dissolved.

For Intravenous Injection: Reconstitute only with Sterile Water for Injection.

Reconstitution Table for Standard Vials – I.V. Injection			
Vial Size	Diluent to be Added to Vial	Approximate Available Volume	Approximate Average Concentration
1 g	10 mL	10.7 mL	95 mg/mL
2 g	20 mL	21.4 mL	95 mg/mL

Shake well until dissolved.

For Intravenous Infusion: Reconstitute as for intravenous injection. Further dilute the reconstituted solution to 50 to 100 mL with one of the "Solutions for Intravenous Infusion" (see below).

Adult Dose Range: 1-12 grams daily in equally divided doses every 8 -12 hours.

Reconstitution:
I.M.: Add **3 mL** Sterile Water for Injection or Bacteriostatic Water for Injection; **shake well**; yields **270 mg** ceftizoxime/mL.
I.V.: Add **10 mL** Sterile Water for Injection; **shake well**; yields **95 mg** ceftizoxime/mL.
I.V. Infusion: Reconstitute as above; further dilute with one of the recommended I.V. infusion solutions. Use reconstituted solution within 24 hours if kept at room temperature or 48 hours if refrigerated.

See Package Insert. Product Monograph available on request. Store powder at room temperature (15°C - 30°C).
under licence of Fujisawa Pharmaceutical Co., Ltd., Osaka, Japan
SmithKline Beecham Pharma Inc.
Oakville, Ontario L6H 5V2

DIN 01919490

℞ CEFIZOX ®
STERILE CEFTIZOXIME SODIUM USP
CEFTIZOXIME SODIQUE STÉRILE USP

1 g ceftizoxime/vial/fiole

ANTIBIOTIC/ANTIBIOTIQUE
For Intramuscular or Intravenous Use
Pour usage intramusculaire ou intraveineux

SB SmithKline Beecham

Posologie pour adultes : 1-12 grammes par jour en doses fractionnées toutes les 8-12 heures.
Reconstitution : Injection i.m. : Ajouter **3 mL** d'eau stérile ou bactériostatique pour injection; **bien agiter;** donne **270 mg** ceftizoxime/mL.
Injection i.v. : Ajouter **10 mL** d'eau stérile pour injection; **bien agiter;** donne **95 mg** ceftizoxime/mL.
Perfusion i.v. : Reconstituer comme ci-dessus, diluer davantage avec l'une des solutions pour perfusion i.v. recommandées. Utiliser la solution reconstituée dans les 24 heures si gardée à la température ambiante ou 48 heures si réfrigérée. Voir notice. Monographie envoyée sur demande. Conserver la poudre à la température ambiante (15 °C - 30 °C).
titulaire d'une licence de Fujisawa Pharmaceutical Co., Ltd., Osaka, Japon

173H971

Label A

Adult Dose Range: 1-12 grams daily in equally divided doses every 8 -12 hours.

Reconstitution:
I.M.: Add **6 mL** Sterile Water for Injection or Bacteriostatic Water for Injection; **shake well**; yields **270 mg** ceftizoxime/mL.
I.V.: Add **20 mL** Sterile Water for Injection; **shake well**; yields **95 mg** ceftizoxime/mL.
I.V. Infusion: Reconstitute as above; further dilute with one of the recommended I.V. infusion solutions. Use reconstituted solution within 24 hours if kept at room temperature or 48 hours if refrigerated.

See Package Insert. Product Monograph available on request. Store powder at room temperature (15°C - 30°C).
under licence of Fujisawa Pharmaceutical Co., Ltd., Osaka, Japan
SmithKline Beecham Pharma Inc.
Oakville, Ontario L6H 5V2

DIN 01919504

℞ CEFIZOX ®
STERILE CEFTIZOXIME SODIUM USP
CEFTIZOXIME SODIQUE STÉRILE USP

2 g ceftizoxime/vial/fiole

ANTIBIOTIC/ANTIBIOTIQUE
For Intramuscular or Intravenous Use
Pour usage intramusculaire ou intraveineux

SB SmithKline Beecham

Posologie pour adultes : 1-12 grammes par jour en doses fractionnées toutes les 8-12 heures.
Reconstitution : Injection i.m. : Ajouter **6 mL** d'eau stérile ou bactériostatique pour injection; **bien agiter;** donne **270 mg** ceftizoxime/mL.
Injection i.v. : Ajouter **20 mL** d'eau stérile pour injection; **bien agiter;** donne **95 mg** ceftizoxime/mL.
Perfusion i.v. : Reconstituer comme ci-dessus, diluer davantage avec l'une des solutions pour perfusion i.v. recommandées. Utiliser la solution reconstituée dans les 24 heures si gardée à la température ambiante ou 48 heures si réfrigérée. Voir notice. Monographie envoyée sur demande. Conserver la poudre à la température ambiante (15 °C - 30 °C).
titulaire d'une licence de Fujisawa Pharmaceutical Co., Ltd., Osaka, Japon

173H981

Label B

4002A/1191

STOOL SOFTENER
Indications: Occasional or temporary constipation.
Daily Oral Dose: Children 6 to 12 years - 1 capsule. Adults and older children - 1 or 2 capsules.
The effect of COLACE* on the stools may not be apparent for one to three days after the first oral dose.
Precautions: Do not use in the presence of abdominal pain, nausea, fever or vomiting. Frequent or prolonged use may result in dependence on laxatives. Do not administer COLACE* within two hours of another medicine, to avoid reduction of its effect.
Keep this and all medication out of the reach of children.

*T.M. Auth. User/Usager autor. de la M.D. Bristol-Myers Squibb Canada Inc.

Do not use if seal is broken
SAFETY SEALED BOTTLE

BRISTOL

Colace*

Docusate Sodium Capsules U.S.P.
Capsules de docusate de sodium U.S.P.
100 mg/capsule
BRISTOL LABORATORIES of Canada
LABORATOIRES BRISTOL du Canada
Division of/de Bristol-Myers Squibb Canada Inc.
Montreal, Canada

100 Capsules
DIN 00464767
LIST/E 320110

MANCHON DE SÉCURITÉ
Ne pas utiliser si le manchon est endommagé

ÉMOLLIENT FÉCAL
Indications: Constipation occasionnelle ou passagère.
Dose orale quotidienne: Enfants de 6 à 12 ans - 1 capsule. Adultes et adolescents - 1 ou 2 capsules.
L'effet de COLACE* sur les selles peut n'être apparent que de 1 à 3 jours après la dose initiale par voie orale.
Précautions: Ne pas utiliser en présence de douleurs abdominales, de nausées, de fièvre ou de vomissements. Son utilisation fréquente ou prolongée peut causer une accoutumance aux laxatifs. Ne pas administrer COLACE* dans les deux heures suivant la prise d'un autre médicament, ce qui pourrait réduire son effet.
Garder ce produit et tout autre médicament hors de la portée des enfants.

Exp.

List

Case Study 3

Mrs. B., age 60, has had chronic lung disease for 3 years and is admitted with pneumonia. IV orders:
NS continuous at 100 mL/h
methylprednisolone (SoluMedrol) 80 mg in 50 mL NS q8h with flow rate of 100 mL/h
ceftizoxime (Cefizox) 2 g in 50 mL D5W q8h and rate of 100 mL/h
Other medication orders include bronchodilators by inhaler and nebulizer and Colace 200 mg PO daily.

---

1. State the generic name for Colace.

2. What is the product form of Colace?

3. What is the product strength of Colace?

4. Calculate the number of capsules for the Colace order.

5. A 50 mL minibag labelled SoluMedrol 80 mg is hung by IVPB at 0800 h. At what time will it be absorbed?

6. What time will the next dose of SoluMedrol be due?

Prepare the IV admixture for Cefizox for 0900 h.

7. Is the ordered dose within the recommended range?

8. Describe the reconstitution (state the product you are using).

9. State the resulting concentration.

10. Calculate the volume to add to the 50 mL minibag of D5W.

11. State the concentration of the IV solution prepared. (Remember, you have added volume to the minibag!)

12. How long is this solution stable?

13. At what time will this dose be absorbed?

14. What time is the next dose of Cefizox due?

15. What is the total volume of IV fluid infused over 24 hours? (Include the primary IV and the minibag volumes.)

16. How much NS does Mrs. B. receive over 24 hours?

17. How much D5W does Mrs. B. receive over 24 hours?

Three days after admission, the intravenous is discontinued and a new order for Cefizox 1 g IM q8h is written.

18. Describe the reconstitution of the Cefizox. Use product label A.

19. State the resulting concentration.

20. Calculate the volume to administer for the above order.

21. Describe the reconstitution if only product label B is available.

22. Using product label B, calculate the volume to administer for the above order.

23. How long is the reconstituted solution stable?

24. How many doses can be given from product label B?

Case Study 4

Preparing medications for several patients.

It is 0745h and you must give medications to 3 patients. Refer to drug labels on page 151. Use this schedule.

        daily: 0800 h
        bid: 0800 h, and 2000 h
        tid: 0800 h, 1600 h, and 2200 h
        hs: 2200 h
        meal times: 0800 h, 1200 h, and 1700 h

Medication Orders

Mr. Ziebart	Mrs. Flanagan	Miss Perman
Capoten 12.5 mg PO daily	Desyrel 50 mg PO am and	Sinemet 100/10 and 250 PO bid
Lasix 20 mg PO bid	75 mg PO hs	Ludiomil 50 mg PO hs
Atasol 15 tab i PO am and hs	digoxin 0.375 mg PO daily	digoxin 0.25 mg PO daily
	lorazepam 0.5 mg PO bid	
	Entrophen 500 mg PO daily	
	Cytotec 0.1 mg PO with meals	

Mr. Ziebart:

Order	Product	Number of tablets
(1)	(2)	(3)
(4)	(5)	(6)
(7)	(8)	(9)

Mrs. Flanagan:

Order	Product	Number of tablets
(10)	(11)	(12)
(13)	(14)	(15)
(16)	(17)	(18)
(19)	(20)	(21)
(22)	(23)	(24)

Miss Perman:

Order	Product	Number of tablets
(25)	(26)	(27)
(28)	(29)	(30)

(A)

Entrophen
325 mg tablets

(B)

Entrophen
0.5 g tablets

(C)

Sinemet
100/10

(D)

Sinemet
250

(E)

maprotiline
25 mg tablets
Ludiomil

(F)

captopril
25 mg tablets
(scored)
Capoten

(G)

misoprostol
100 mcg tablets
Cytotec

(H)

furosemide
20 mg tablets
Lasix

(I)

acetaminophen
325 mg
codeine 15 mg
caffeine 15 mg
Atasol 15

(J)

digoxin
250 mcg tablets
Lanoxin

(K)

digoxin
0.125 mg tablets
Lanoxin

(L)

trazodone HCL
100 mg tablets
Desyrel

(M)

trazodone HCL
50 mg tablets
Desyrel

(N)

lorazepam
0.5 mg tablets
Ativan

(O)

lorazepam
1 mg tablets
Ativan

Case Study 5

Mrs. Oma, 59-years-old, is admitted with severe pain due to exacerbation of sickle cell disease. Orders:
morphine IV 5 mg/h and 5 mg IM q2h for breakthrough pain. For each IM dose, increase IV rate by 1 mg/h
Drug supplied as 200mg/500 mL lactated Ringer's. Use an infusion pump.
IV initiated at 2300 h.

---

1.   Calculate initial IV infusion rate.

2.   At 0115 h, 5 mg IM is required for breakthrough pain. Calculate the adjusted IV rate.

3.   At 0345 h, 5 mg IM is required for breakthrough pain. Calculate new infusion rate.

4.   At 0545 h, another IM dose of 5 mg is administered. What should the IV rate be?

5.   By 0700 h Mrs. Oma is comfortable. No further IM doses are required. Calculate the total amount of morphine received from 2300 h to 0700 h.

Case Study 6

John is newly diagnosed with diabetes mellitus. He is 32-years-old, married, with one child. He attends the day program to learn to monitor his blood glucose and adjust his insulin doses accordingly. He does a blood glucose test before each meal and at hs. The insulin orders are:
If blood glucose

< 10 mmol/L,   0 units of Humulin R
< 15 mmol/L,   5 units of Humulin R
< 20 mmol/L,   8 units of Humulin R
< 30 mmol/L,   10 units of Humulin R

Complete the table on the following page.

Study the table and add the correct dose for each blood glucose reading.

Time	Blood glucose	Insulin dose
ac breakfast	9.7 (mmol/L)	(1)
ac lunch	21.5	(2)
ac supper	12.9	(3)
hs	4.6	(4)
ac breakfast	9.9	(5)
ac lunch	15.4	(6)
ac supper	13.8	(7)
hs	9.7	(8)

9.   Shade the syringe to show the dosage given ac lunch on first day.

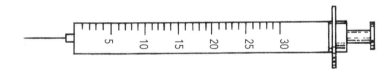

10. Calculate the total amount of insulin received each day.

Module 9: Calculations for Children and Critical Care

Module Topics

- calculating dosages for children
- calculations based on body weight
- titrating intravenous and medications
- using calculation tables
- case studies
- posttest

Introduction

In every clinical situation involving medication administration, accurate dosage calculation is an important responsibility. Neonatal, paediatric, elderly, and acutely-ill patients require very precise dosage administration. This module does not present any new mathematic principles but does provide practice in more complex dosage calculations, using body weight and dosages titrated by the IV route.

Calculating Dosages for Children

Today, most references indicate the recommended dosages for children. For adults standard dosage ranges exist, but for children, because of the many factors of age, body weight, and disease factors, the dose is often stated as amount to give per kg of body weight. This requires additional steps of calculation.

> **CRITICAL POINT**
>
> It is a nursing responsibility to calculate and validate the dosage calculation and also to confirm that the dose is within the recommended range. Dosage errors can be very serious for infants/children. Develop the habit of always writing your calculation and asking a colleague to validate.

Calculations Based on Body Weight

Frequently, a dose for a child is written as "amount of drug per kg of body weight," e.g., 1 mg/kg q6h. The dose may also be stated as an amount to give in 24 hours in a specific number of divided doses. The following example illustrates the steps of calculations based on the body weight and the procedure for confirmation, calculation, and validation of the dose for children.

1. Determine the recommended dose from a reliable literature source (text, package insert, or pharmacy literature).

   e.g., child 12 years, penicillin G 200 000 units per kg per day in equally divided doses q4–6h.

2. Compare the recommended and the prescribed dose. In the example, the dose is within the recommended range.

   order: penicillin G 200 000 units/kg/day q6h

3. Calculate the dose for a 9-year-old child, 32 kg.

   200 000 U × 32 kg = 6 400 000 U/day q6h = 4 doses = 1 600 000 U per dose (or 1.6 million units).

4. Calculate the dose to administer. Vial label states 5 million units (5 m U) Label instructions: add 3.1 mL diluent to yield a volume of 5 mL.

   Use proportion:
   5m U : 5 mL = 1.6 m U : x mL
   x mL = 1.6 mL.

5. Validate.

   5 m U : 5 mL = 1.6 m U : 1.6 mL.

In some situations, the physician may order the specific dose to be given for each administration. The steps are similar to the previous example. Let's do another example.

1. Determine the recommended dose from a reliable source.

   cefuroxime 50–100 mg/kg/day divided q6–8h.

2. Compare the recommended and prescribed doses.

   order: cefuroxime 860 mg IV q8h.

3. Calculate the dose for 12-year-old, weight 34.5 kg.

   860 mg × 3 doses = 2 580 mg/day; per kg dose is 2 580/34.5 = 74.78 mg/kg (rounded to 75 mg/kg).

Conclusion

75 mg/kg is within range of 50–100 mg/kg

Exercise 9.1

For additional practice with dosages for children based on body weight, complete this exercise. (Value: 1 each).
Round oral dosages to the nearest whole number.
Round parenteral doses to the nearest hundredth.

Recommended dose for a child < 10-years-old, 4 mg/kg/day in 4 equally divided doses not to exceed 200 mg/day. Recommended dose for a child > 10 or adults, 5 mg/kg/day in 4 equally divided doses not to exceed 400 mg/day.

1. Michael is 9-years-old and weighs 20 kg. Calculate the recommended daily dose.

2. Calculate each of Michael's doses.

3. Mary is 14-years-old and weighs 51.2 kg. Calculate her recommended daily dose.

4. Confirm whether Mary's dose is within the recommended range.

Order #2: erythromycin 345 mg PO q6h. Recommended dose is 20–50 mg/kg/day in 4 divided doses.

5. Calculate the total daily dose for Jennifer.

6. Jennifer is 11-years-old and weighs 34.5 kg. Confirm whether Jennifer's dose is within the recommended range.

7. The erythromycin is supplied in a suspension labelled 125 mg/5 mL. Calculate the amount that must be administered for each dose.

Order #3: Tylenol Elixir PO q4h prn for pain. The recommended dose for a child < 10 years old, is 10–15 mg/kg/dose, not to exceed 65 mg/kg/day, and for an adult or child > 10-years-old, 325–650 mg q4h prn, not to exceed 4 g per day.

8. What is the safe dosage range for Colleen, age 7-years-old and weighing 22.5 kg?

9. An order is written for Jennifer (question #2) for 480 mg PO q4h. Is this within the recommended range?

10. James, age 3 years, weight 12.6 kg, is ordered 100 mg. Is this dose acceptable?

11. The Tylenol Elixir label states 160 mg/5mL. Calculate the dose in mL for Patricia, age 4 years, weight 17 kg, if the order is for 10 mg/kg.

Order #4: Kate is 1-year-old, weighs 13 lbs and is ordered a loading dose of IV digoxin 175 mcg. The literature states that the loading (initial) dose for a child < 2-years-old is 0.015–0.035 mg/kg administered IV over 5 minutes. The maintenance dose is 25% of the digitalizing dose.

12. Is Kate's loading dose within the recommended range?

13. If digoxin is supplied in an ampule labelled "250 mcg/mL," calculate the volume for Kate's initial IV dose.

14. Determine Kate's maintenance oral dose. Calculate how much to administer if the digoxin elixir is labelled 50 mcg/mL.

Order #5: The recommended dose for SoluMedrol is 0.5–1 mg/kg/dose given q6h.

15. SoluMedrol 8.5 mg IV q6h is ordered for Stacy, age 4-years-old, weight 17 kg. Is this dose within the recommendations?

16. SoluMedrol is available in an ampule labelled 20 mg/mL. Calculate the volume required for Stacy's dose.

17. What is the total dose of SoluMedrol administered to Stacy in 24 hours?

Order #6: Recommended dose for epinephrine is 0.01 mL of 1:1 000 solution per kg as a single dose. Available: epinephrine 1:1 000 solution (or 1 mg/mL).

18. Lara weighs 15 kg and is ordered 10 mcg/kg epinephrine SC stat. Is this within the recommended range?

19. Calculate how much to administer using the above supply of epinephrine.

20. Shade in the dose on the syringe.

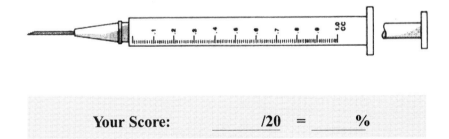

Your Score: _____ **/20** = _____ **%**

Exercise 9.2

Assume that all the orders are confirmed within the recommended range. Calculate the dose in mg and the volume of drug product to administer. Correct using the answer guide. (Value: 2 each, 1 point for calculation and 1 point for rounding). Round oral dosages to the nearest whole number. Round parenteral doses to the nearest hundredth.

1. A child weighing 17 kg is to receive 5 mg/kg PO of an antibiotic. A syrup labelled 25 mg/ mL is available.

2. A child weighing 11.5 kg is to receive a dose of erythromycin 10 mg/kg PO. Medication containing 125 mg/5 mL is available.

3. The order states: 0.015 mg/kg loading dose of digoxin IV. Calculate the volume required for this dose for a child weighing 3.2 kg if the available strength is 0.25 mg/mL.

4. Is this order safe? The preoperative order for a 10-year-old boy who weighs 34 kg is for atropine sulfate 0.01 mg/kg IM 1 hour preoperatively. The literature states that 0.4 mg is the maximum dose that may be given to a child.

5. The order states: Phenobarb 2 mg/kg PO bid. Calculate the dose in mL for a child weighing 19 lbs. Available strength is 15 mg/5 mL.

6. The infant's weight is 3.9 kg; the order is for Lasix 2 mg/kg IV. Lasix 10 mg/mL is available.

7. The infant's order is gentamicin 2 mg IV q12h. Gentamicin 20 mg/2 mL is available.

8. The infant's weight is 11.2 kg and the order is for ampicillin 50 mg/kg/day IV q6h in equally divided doses. Ampicillin 125 mg/mL in a 2 mL vial is available.

9. The infant's weight is 860 g, and the order is for morphine 0.6 mg/kg/day SC in 6 divided doses. Calculate each dose in mg. Calculate the volume to give if the drug is supplied as 2 mg/mL.

10. Alice is a 9-month-old who weighs 7.2 kg. She has received acetaminophen 60 mg PO q4h × 24 hours. The literature states that a child < 1 year should receive 15–60 mg/dose q4–6h not to exceed 65 mg/kg/day. Has she received more than the daily limit?

Your Score: _____ **/20** = _____ **%**

Paediatric Case Study

Complete this case study to practice using package insert literature.

> Sean weighs 32 pounds and is to receive Ancef, 25 mg/kg/day in 3 equal doses.

Use the table from the package insert of Ancef (cefazolin sodium) below to answer the questions.

1. What is the frequency of administration for this order?

2. What is the approximate single dose in mg?

3. What volume is needed to deliver this dose?

4. How is the powder reconstituted to produce a concentration of 125 mg/mL?

Calculate the following without referring to the package insert and compare your responses with the previous answers.

5. Based on body weight, what total daily dose would Sean receive?

6. How much should he receive for each dose of Ancef?

7. Compare answers for #2 and #6: explain the difference.

8. Refer again to the package insert: what volume should Sean receive if the frequency is changed to qid?

PEDIATRIC DOSAGE GUIDE - 25 mg/kg/day

Weight		25 mg/kg/day Divided into 3 Doses		25 mg/kg/day Divided into 4 Doses	
lb	kg	Approximate Single Dose mg/q8h	Volume Needed of 125 mg/mL* Solution	Approximate Single Dose mg/q6h	Volume Needed of 125 mg/mL* Solution
10	4.5	40 mg	0.35 mL	30 mg	0.25 mL
20	9.0	75 mg	0.60 mL	55 mg	0.45 mL
30	13.6	115 mg	0.90 mL	85 mg	0.70 mL
40	18.1	150 mg	1.20 mL	115 mg	0.90 mL
50	22.7	190 mg	1.50 mL	140 mg	1.10 mL

*125 mg/mL concentration may be obtained by reconstituting the 500 mg vial with 3.8 mL of diluent.

PEDIATRIC DOSAGE GUIDE - 50 mg/kg/day

Weight		50 mg/kg/day Divided into 3 Doses		50 mg/kg/day Divided into 4 Doses	
lb	kg	Approximate Single Dose mg/q8h	Volume Needed of 225 mg/mL* Solution	Approximate Single Dose mg/q6h	Volume Needed of 225 mg/mL* Solution
10	4.5	75 mg	0.35 mL	55 mg	0.25 mL
20	9.0	150 mg	0.70 mL	110 mg	0.50 mL
30	13.6	225 mg	1.00 mL	170 mg	0.75 mL
40	18.1	300 mg	1.35 mL	225 mg	1.00 mL
50	22.7	375 mg	1.70 mL	285 mg	1.25 mL

*225 mg/mL solution may be obtained by reconstituting the 500 mg vial with 2.0 mL of diluent.

Titrating Intravenous Medications

Dosages in critical care and emergency units are usually calculated by titration, that is, the dose is frequently adjusted to the patient's condition. The dose often will be ordered as a weight or volume of drug per kilogram of body weight per unit of time, for example, 5 mcg/kg/minute.

Drugs used in these settings are potent, and the flow rate must be carefully and accurately monitored. The drugs are delivered by intravenous piggyback (IVPB), a volutrol or buretrol chamber in the infusion line, and direct IV push. To achieve accuracy, it is safest to use a regulating machine to control the rate of flow and an infusion set that delivers 60 drops/minute (a microdrip set).

The following are two exercises that present opportunities to practice titrating medications. The first focuses on neonates in critical care; the second involves adults in critical care or emergency settings. These calculations require a careful, step-by-step approach. You should write out the problem and the solution, then validate your answer. In many instances, nurses are expected to write the calculations directly on the patient's record and validate their answers with a colleague. To calculate the rate of flow of IV medications, you can solve step-by-step using ratio and proportion, or you can use the formula.

Calculation Formula

To determine flow rate for mcg/kg/minute (expressed in mL/h):

$$\frac{\text{mcg required x weight (kg)} \times 60 \text{ minutes/hour}}{\text{concentration (mcg per mL)}} = \underline{\hspace{1cm}} \text{ mL/h}$$

Example:

Give dopamine 5 mcg/kg/minute.
Patient weighs 61 kg.

Mix 200 mg in 250 mL:
Concentration = 200 ÷ 250 = 0.8 mg = 800 mcg per mL

$$\frac{5 \text{ mcg} \times 61 \text{ kg} \times 60 \text{ min}}{800 \text{ mcg per mL}} = 22.875 \text{ mL/hour}$$

Run at 23 mL/hour = 23 drops per minute (minidrip)

NOTE: This formula can also be used to calculate an order for mg/kg/h. Simply substitute mg for mcg.

Let's do another example. Nurses in some settings have devised flow charts or other helpful tools to assist with these calculations, which often vary in response to changes in a patient's parameters. Examples of these tools are also included in this module. Let's use the tool in the box to calculate a dopamine drip.

Formula for Mixing Dopamine Solution

To make 50 mL of solution that provides 5 mcg/kg/minute at a rate of 1 mL/hour:

(5 mcg × _____ kg × 60 minutes × 50 mL = _____ mcg dopamine in 50 mL of IV solution
_____ mcg ÷ 40 000 mcg/mL =_____ mL dopamine

Dopamine Drip

Using the solution concentration determined above, the nurse can adjust the IV rate in mL/hour as follows:

IV rate	Dopamine dosage
0.5 mL/hour	2.5 mcg/kg/minute
1 mL/hour	5 mcg/kg/minute
1.5 mL/hour	7.5 mcg/kg/minute

Example:

Infant's weight: 860 g or 0.86 kg
Order: Dopamine 5 mcg/kg/minute in D5W at 1 mL/hour

Solution:
To make 50 mL of solution that provides 5 mcg/kg/minute at a rate of 1 mL/hour:

(5 mcg × 0.86 × 60 minutes × 50 mL) =
12 900 mcg dopamine in 50 mL of IV solution

View label on page 162 and note the available concentration of dopamine: convert to mcg.

40 mg/mL = 40 000 mcg/mL

Calculate the dose of dopamine.

12 900 mcg ÷ 40 000 mcg/mL = 0.32 mL dopamine

Prepare the IV solution and run at 1 mL per hour to provide 5 mcg/kg/minute.

EXP ⊓ LOT	NDC 0641-**0112-25** 25 x **5 mL** *Single Use* Vials **DOPAMINE** HCl INJECTION, USP **200 mg/5 mL** (40 mg/mL) FOR IV INFUSION ONLY	**POTENT DRUG: MUST DILUTE BEFORE USING** Each mL contains dopamine hydrochloride 40 mg (equivalent to 32.3 mg dopamine base) and sodium bisulfite 10 mg in Water for Injection. pH 2.5-5.0. Sealed under nitrogen. USUAL DOSE: See package insert. Do not use if solution is discolored. Store at 15° - 30° C (59° - 86° F). Caution: Federal law prohibits dispensing without prescription. B-50112c

⊖Si ELKINS-SINN, INC. Cherry Hill, NJ 08003-4099
A subsidiary of A H Robins Company

Using Calculation Tables

To assist clinicians with complex calculations, some settings use dosage tables. Read the Dopamine Dosage Table and the examples and then try Exercise 9.3.

Dopamine Dosage Table

Add 200 mg to 500 mL solution.
Concentration: 400 mcg/mL solution

> Find body weight across the top.
> Find desired dose on left side.
> Follow line across table to determine flow rate in mL/hour
> (or drops per minute using a minidrip set with a drop factor of 60
>   drops = 1 mL).

mcg/min	Body Weight (in kg)									
	50	55	60	65	70	75	80	85	90	95
1	7	8	9	10	11	11	12	13	13	14
2	15	17	18	19	21	23	24	25	27	29
3	23	23	27	29	31	34	36	38	41	43
4	30	33	36	39	42	45	48	51	54	57
5	37	41	45	49	53	56	60	64	67	71

Examples:
Patient weighs 65 kg.
Order: 2 mcg/minute
Rate is 19 mL/h (or 19 gtts/min).

Find 65 on top line
Find 2 on left side

Patient weighs 69 kg.
Order: 4 mcg/minute
Rate is 42 mL/h (or 42 gtts/min).

Closest number is 70 kg
Find 4 on left side

Patient weighs 75 kg.
Order: 3.5 mcg/minute

Find 75 on top line
Find rates for 3 and 4: Rate for 3 is 34
mL/h and rate for 4 is 45 mL/h:
find midpoint = 39.5 (approx. 40 mL/h)

These examples can be validated with the formula.

$$\frac{\text{mcg required} \times \text{weight (kg)} \times 60 \text{ min/h}}{\text{mcg per mL}} = \text{mL/h}$$

$$\frac{2 \times 65 \times 60}{400} = (19.5) = 20 \text{ mL/h}$$

$$\frac{4 \times 69 \times 60}{400} = (41.4) = 41 \text{ mL/h}$$

$$\frac{3.5 \times 75 \times 60}{400} = (39.3) = 39 \text{ mL/h}$$

Exercise 9.3

Calculate the following problems. For each situation, write the problem and solution and then validate your answers. Round decimal numbers to the nearest hundredth.

1. An infant weighing 600 g is to receive gentamicin sulfate (Garamycin) 2.5 mg/kg by IV infusion q12h. The drug is supplied in a concentration of 10 mg/mL. Calculate the volume of drug to add to the IV fluid.

    Order: An infant weighing 11 lbs must receive a loading dose of aminophylline 7.5 mg/kg by IV infusion over 20 minutes. This is to be followed by maintenance doses of 0.5 mg/kg/h by continuous IV infusion. The drug is available in 50 mg/5 mL ampule.

2. Calculate the loading dose for the order above.

3. Calculate the amount of drug to add to a 25 mL IV minibag to produce a concentration of 1 mg/mL for the order above.

4. Calculate the rate of flow for the maintenance dose for the order above.

5. An isoproterenol drip is running at 1 mL/hour and delivers 2 mcg/kg/minute. The infant weighs 1 265 grams. How much drug does the infant receive each hour?

Use the formula below for questions 6-10.

Formula for Mixing Dopamine Solution

To make 50 mL of solution that provides 5 mcg/kg/minute at a rate of 1 mL/ hour:

(5 mcg/kg/minute × _____ kg × 60 minutes × 50 mL = _____ mcg dopamine in 50 mL of IV solution

_____ mcg ÷ 40 000 mcg/mL = _____ mL dopamine

IV rate	Dopamine dosage
0.5 mL/hour	2.5 mcg/kg/minute
1 mL/hour	5 mcg/kg/minute
1.5 mL/hour	7.5 mcg/kg/minute

---

6. An infant's weight is 790 g. The order is for dopamine 5 mcg/kg/minute. Calculate the amount of dopamine to add to a 50 mL IV solution.

    5 mcg × _____ kg × 60 minutes × 50 mL = _____ mcg dopamine in 50 mL.

    _____ mcg/40 000 mcg/mL = _____ mL dopamine

7. Determine the rate of flow from the chart above.

8. State the IV rate necessary to deliver 2.5 mcg/kg/minute.

9. The infant's weight is 1170 g. The order is for dopamine 7.5 mcg/kg/minute. Determine the amount of dopamine required to prepare the solution.

10. Determine the amount of dopamine received in 1 hour.

Your Score: _____ /10 = _____ %

Exercise 9.4

Read the label on the IV bag. Use the calculation formula and solve these situations.

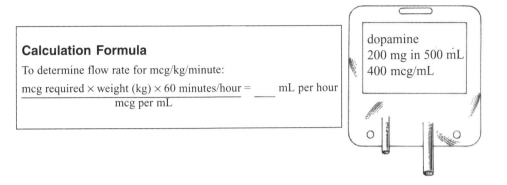

Calculation Formula

To determine flow rate for mcg/kg/minute:

$$\frac{\text{mcg required} \times \text{weight (kg)} \times 60 \text{ minutes/hour}}{\text{mcg per mL}} = \underline{\quad} \text{ mL per hour}$$

dopamine
200 mg in 500 mL
400 mcg/mL

Determine the rate of flow in mL/hour. (Express as whole number)

1) Dopamine 3 mcg/kg/min for patient weighing 52 kg.

2) Dopamine 4 mcg/kg/min for patient weighing 64 kg.

3) Dopamine 6 mcg/kg/min for patient weighing 77 kg.

4) Dopamine 5 mcg/kg/min for patient weighing 75 kg.

5) Dopamine 8 mcg/kg/min for patient weighing 178 lbs.

Your Score: _____ /5 = _____ %

Exercise 9.5
(Value: 1 each answer).

1. State the concentration of medication in mcg per mL if 400 mg of drug is added to 500 mL of IV solution.

2. Prepare an intravenous solution of 250 mg of medication in 250 mL of solution. State the concentration of mcg/mL.

3. Using an IV solution concentration of 1 mg/250 mL, calculate the rate of flow in mL/hour to deliver 3.5 mcg/minute.

4. Calculate the rate of infusion in mL/h for: dopamine 3 mcg/kg/minute for a patient weighing 70 kg. Use a minibag containing 200 mg in 250 mL.

Order: give 2 mcg/kg/minute IV. Answer questions 5 through 7.

5. Calculate the dose required per hour for a patient weighing 65 kg.

6. Calculate the concentration (in mcg/mL) if 200 mg drug in 250 mL IV.

7. Calculate the rate of flow in mL/h.

8. An IV minibag admixture is prepared with 1 mg of isoproterenol in 250 mL of solution. What is the concentration in mcg/mL?

9. If 50 mg of a drug is added to 250 mL of IV solution, how much of the drug does the patient receive per minute at a rate of 60 mL/h?

Epinephrine Hydrocloride (Adrenaline) Concentration Table

Prepare the appropriate concentration by mixing the indicated amount of drug in the volume of IV solution. Select the dose in mcg per minute in the left column. Follow the line across the table to determine the rate of flow in mL per hour (or drops per minute using a minidrip set with a drop factor of 60 drops = 1 mL).

Dose (mcg/minute)	1 mg/250 mL (4 mcg/mL)	4 mg/500 ml (8 mcg/mL)	2.5 mg/250 mL (10 mcg/mL)
0.5	7	4	—
1	15	8	6
2	30	15	12
3	45	23	18
4	60	30	24
5	75	38	30
6	90	45	36

Refer to the epinephrine concentration table for questions 10, 11, and 12.

10. The concentration of the epinephrine solution is 4 mcg/mL. State:
    a. the number of mg in 250 mL of IV solution.
    b. the rate of flow necessary to deliver 2 mcg/minute.
    c. how many mcg are delivered in 15 minutes if the rate of flow is 45 drops/minute.

11. State:
    a. the concentration of the epinephrine solution in mcg/mL if 4 mg were added to 500mL.
    b. the flow rate required to deliver 1 mcg/minute.
    c. how many mcg/minute the patient is receiving if the IV pump is set at 23 mL/hour.

12. A 250 mL bag is labelled "1 mg epinephrine added."
    (a) What is the dose in mcg/minute if the rate is 15 mL/h?
    (b) What rate is required to deliver 3 mcg/minute?
    (c) The IV is running at 30 mL/h for 30 minutes.
        How much (total) epinephrine has the patient received?
    (d) The order states "Run epinephrine at 4 mcg/minute." The IV pump is set for 30 mL/h.
        Is this correct?
    (e) The patient has received 200 mL. How much epinephrine has been given?

Your Score: _____ **/20** = _____ **%**

Case Studies

Read the case studies then calculate the volume required and product for all medications ordered. Refer to the boxes on pages 168 and 169.

Case Study 1

Mr. M., age 55, is admitted complaining of chest pain. Telemetry showed short runs of multifocal PVCs followed by ventricular fibrillation. CPR was commenced and IV initiated (with a minidrip set).
Orders:

lidocaine 100 mg IV bolus
lidocaine commenced 4 mg/minute
Pronestyl 1 g IV bolus
lidocaine drip discontinued
Pronestyl drip at 4 mg/minute
calcium gluconate 1 ampule

---

1. Lidocaine bolus.
2. Lidocaine drip: describe preparation.
3. Lidocaine drip: state flow rate.
4. Pronestyl bolus.
5. Pronestyl drip: describe preparation.
6. Pronestyl drip: state flow rate.

Case Study 2

A middle-aged man in the CCU is monitored; he weighs 71 kg. An IV is running with a minidrip set and volumetric pump. Respiratory arrest and ventricular tachycardia occur. Orders:

· lidocaine 100 mg IV bolus
Xylocaine drip 1 mg/minute
dopamine drip 3 mcg/kg/minute

---

7. Xylocaine drip: describe preparation and state flow rate.
8. Lasix bolus.

Case Study 3

Mrs. T. was admitted by ambulance to the C.C.U. She was short of breath and experiencing retrosternal chest pain radiating to the jaw. Orders:

Isuprel drip 2 mcg/minute

---

9. Isuprel drip; state preparation and flow rate.
10. Increase drip to 2.5 mcg/minute.

Emergency Medications

Drug	Strength	Volume (ampule or vial)
dopamine (Intropin)	40 mg/mL	5 mL ampule
furosemide (Lasix)	10 mg/mL	4 mL ampule
isoproterenol HCl (Isuprel)	1 mg/5 mL	5 mL ampule
lidocaine HCl (Xylocaine)	20 mg/mL	5 mL ampule
lidocaine HCl (Xylocaine)	1 g/50 mL	50 mL vial
procainamide HCl (Pronestyl)	100 mg/mL	5 mL ampule

Lidocaine (Xylocaine) Drip

Add 2 g to 500 mL D5W: use a minidrip set (60 drops/mL)

1 mg/minute = 15 mL/hour
2 mg/minute = 30 mL/hour
3 mg/minute = 45 mL/hour
4 mg/minute = 60 mL/hour

Procainamide (Pronestyl) Drip

Add 2 g to 500 mL = 4 mg per mL

1 mg/minute = 15 drops/minute
2 mg/minute = 30 drops/minute
3 mg/minute = 45 drops/minute
4 mg/minute = 60 drops/minute

Isoproterenol HCl (Isuprel) Drip

Add 2 mg to 500 mL IV solution = concentration of 4 mcg/mL

1 mcg/minute = 15 drops/minute
2 mcg/minute = 30 drops/minute
3 mcg/minute = 45 drops/minute
4 mcg/minute = 60 drops/minute

POSTTEST

Instructions

Write the posttest without referring to any reference materials. Express decimal numbers to the nearest hundredth.

Correct the posttest using the answer guide. (Value: 2 each).

If your score is 100 percent, congratulations! You have completed the final module.

If you don't achieve 100 percent, review the learning package in this module and rewrite the posttest.

1. The drug reference book states that 25 mg/kg of Drug T is an appropriate dose. The patient weighs 35 kg. Calculate the recommended dosage.

2. Is the following dosage within the recommended guidelines? A child weighing 15 kg is ordered Drug M 150 mg PO. The literature suggests 6 to 12 mg/kg of this drug for children.

3. An individual who weighs 70 kg is receiving 250 mg of Drug G PO tid. The recommended dose of this drug is 15 mg/kg/day. Is this patient receiving the recommended dose?

4. Calculate the dose to be administered:
     Ordered: 10 mg/kg PO
     Drug available: 200 mg tabs
     Patient weight: 60 kg
     Dose:

5. Calculate the dose to be administered:
     Ordered: 2 mcg/kg IV bolus
     Drug available: 400 mcg/mL
     Patient weight: 50 kg
     Dose:

6. Calculate the dose to administer:
     Ordered: 2 mg/kg
     Drug strength available: 150 mg/mL
     Patient weight: 154 lbs
     Dose:

7. A child weighing 31.5 kg has received too much narcotic, and the antagonist naloxone is ordered: 0.01 mg/kg IM stat. Calculate the dose in mg.

8. For the order in #7, calculate the volume to administer if naloxone is supplied as Narcan 0.4 mg/mL for injection.

9. Order: 30 mg/kg PO daily in 3 doses. Patient weighs 65 kg. Calculate the number of mg for each dose.

10. Order: 10 mg/kg IV q6h and patient weighs 55 kg. Calculate the volume to add to the IV if the available strength is 1 g/mL.

Order #1: 21 mcg/kg/minute IV.

11. For order #1, calculate the dose required for a patient weighing 63 kg.

12. For order #1, if the IV solution contains 1 mg/mL, calculate the rate of flow in gtts/min to deliver the correct dose for a patient weighing 60 kg. The administration set delivers 60 drops/mL.

13. An IV is infusing at 15 gtts/min (the drop factor is 60). The concentration of drug is 80 mg in 100 mL of fluid. How much drug, in mcg, is infusing each minute?

14. A child, age 9 and weight 33 kg, is admitted to emergency with prolonged seizures. Literature recommends dose of 0.3 mg/kg of diazepam (Valium). The ampule label states 10 mg/2 mL. What is the recommended dose for this child?

15. Order for cortisone 10 mg/kg/4 divided doses IV. Calculate a single dose in mg for child weighing 21.2 kg.

Order #2: A patient on a respirator is ordered gallamine tirethiodide (Flaxedil) 1 mg/kg by continuous IV infusion. Calculate the volume required for the dose for a patient weighing 78 kg using the available strengths in 16 and 17 below.

16. A 1 mL ampule containing 100 mg/mL.

17. A 10 mL vial containing 20 mg/mL.

Order #3: dopamine (Intropin) is ordered at 3 mcg/kg/minute. Answer questions 18 and 19 for a patient weighing 79 kg.

18. What is the required dose?

19. If the IV fluid contains 1 mg/mL of dopamine, calculate the rate of infusion in drops/minute using a microdrip (factor of 60 gtts/mL).

20. Calculate the rate of infusion in drops/minute for the same patient but at a new order of 3.5 mg/kg/minute.

Your Score: _____ /40 = _____ %

Appendix: Sample Examinations for Clinical Instructors

The sample examinations were developed for clinical instructors; consequently no answers are provided. Each examination appears in two formats, one with open questions and an identical examination with a multiple-choice format.

These examinations illustrate a comprehensive test of arithmetic skills with whole numbers, fractions, decimal numbers, use of ratio and proportion, understanding systems of measurement, reading medication labels, and calculating oral and parenteral medications. Nursing students should achieve a perfect score on these examinations or review appropriate sections of the book. The examinations can be used in the clinical setting to assess nursing students' skills before medication administration. The examinations are also useful for periodic reevaluation of students' skills.

Examination 1

1. $57\ 809 + 3\ 740 =$
2. $6\ 732 - 599 =$
3. $0.76 \times 1.95 =$
4. $0.25 \div 0.125 =$

5. $\dfrac{1}{3} \times \dfrac{4}{9} =$

6. $\dfrac{7}{15} \div \dfrac{1}{2} =$

7. Which of the following abbreviations means that a drug is to be administered before meals?
   a. ac
   b. pc
   c. hs
8. How many grams are equivalent to 35 mg?
9. The IV order states: infuse 2 000 mL/day. Using a minidrip set (with a drop factor of 60 drops/mL), calculate the rate of flow in mL/hour and drops/minute.
10. How many mL of solution are in the syringe below?

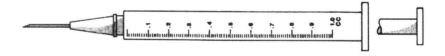

11. The drug is available in 500 mg tablets. How many tablets are required for a dose of 1.5 g?
12. The vial label states NPH insulin 100 units/mL. How many units are contained in 0.4 mL?
13. The order is for 450 000 units of penicillin G and the label states that there are 300 000 units/mL. What amount is required?
14. The label on the penicillin states: 500 000 units/mL. How many units are found in 2.8 mL?

15. The order is for 250 mg of tetracycline. The medication is supplied as a syrup with the concentration of 125 mg/5 mL.
    a. How many mL are required?
    b. How many tsp are required?
16. Which of the following tablets provides the smallest amount of medication?
    a. 0.1 mg
    b. 0.05 mg
    c. 0.15 mg
17. The order reads: 75 mg IM stat.
    Available is a 2 mL ampule with solution concentration of 50 mg/mL.
    How many mL should be given?
18. Ordered: Drug New 15 mg PO in three divided doses. Available: Drug New 2.5 mg tab.
    a. State the amount to administer for each dose.
    b. How many tablets are required for the daily dose?
19. An IV that is infusing at 125 mL/hour has been running for 3 hours and 25 minutes. How much solution should have been infused?
20. Two hundred milligrams of a drug is added to 250 mL of IV solution. What is the concentration in mcg/mL?

Examination 2

1.   57 809 + 3 740 =
     a. 61 549
     b. 62 549
     c. 61 539

2.   6 732 − 599 =
     a. 5 133
     b. 6 133
     c. 6 123

3. $0.76 \times 1.95 =$
     a. 1.482
     b. 14.82
     c. 0.148 2

4. $0.25 \div 0.125 =$
     a. 5
     b. 0.5
     c. 2

5.   1/3 x 4/9 =

     a. $\dfrac{4}{27}$ b. $\dfrac{9}{12}$ c. $\dfrac{3}{4}$

6. $7/15 \div 1/2 =$

     a. $\dfrac{7}{30}$ b. $\dfrac{14}{30}$ c. $\dfrac{14}{15}$

7. Which of the following abbreviations means that a drug is to be administered before meals?
    a. ac
    b. pc
    c. hs

8. How many grams are equivalent fo 35 mg?
    a. 0.035
    b. 0.35
    c. 350

9. The IV order states: infuse 2 000 mL/day. Using a minidrip set (with a drop factor of 60 drops/mL), calculate the rate of flow in mL/hour.
    a. 33 mL/hour
    b. 83 mL/hour
    c. 125 mL/hour

10. How many mL of solution are in the syringe below?
    a. 0.62
    b. 0.6

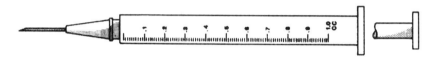

11. The drug is available in 500 mg tablets. How many tablets are required for a dose of 1.5 g?
    a. 3
    b. 2
    c. 2.5

12. The vial label states NPH insulin 100 units/mL. How many units are contained in 0.4 mL?
    a. 4
    b. 40
    c. 400

13. The order is for 450 000 units of penicillin G and the label states that there are 300 000 units/mL. What amount is required?
    a. 1.5 units
    b. 0.67 mL
    c. 1.5 mL

14. The label on the penicillin states: 500 000 units/mL. How many units are found in 2.8 mL?
    a. 1.4 million units
    b. 178 571 units
    c. 140 000 units

15. The order is for 250 mg of tetracycline. The medication is supplied as a syrup with the concentration of 125 mg/5 mL. How many mL are required?
    a. 2 mL
    b. 10 mL
    c. 2.5 mL

11. The drug is available in 250 mg tablets. How many tablets are requried for a dose of 0.5 g?

12. The vial label states: regular insulin 100 units/mL. How many units are contained in 0.34 mL.?

13. The order is for 750 000 units of penicillin G; the label states that there are 300 000 units/mL. How many mL are required?

14. The label on the penicillin states: 1 000 000 units/mL. How many units are found in 2.3 mL?

15. The order is for 12.5 mg. The medication is supplied as a syrup with the concentration of 25 mg/5 mL.
    a. How many mL are required?
    b. How many tsp are required?

16. Which of the following tablets provides the largest amount of medication?
    a. 0.1 mg
    b. 0.05 mg
    c. 0.15 mg

17. The order: 45 mg IM stat. Available: a 2 mL ampule with solution concentration of 50 mg/mL. How many mL should be given?

18. Ordered: Theo-Dur 900 mg PO in 3 divided doses. Available: 300 mg tablets.
    a. What is the amount to administer for each dose?
    b. How many tablets are required for the daily dose?

19. A 1 L bag of IV solution is infusing at 75 mL/hour and has been running for 3 hours and 30 minutes.
    a. How much solution should have been infused?
    b. How much solution should remain?

20. Two hundred milligrams of a drug is added to 500 mL of IV solution. What is the concentration in mcg/mL?

Examination 3

1. 34 989 + 3 450 =
    a. 38 529
    b. 38 439
    c. 38 349

2. 9 345 – 209 =
   a. 9 136
   b. 9 036
   c. 9 055

3. 0.06 × 4.67 =
   a. 0.028 02
   b. 2.802
   c. 0.280 2

4. 0.05 ÷ 0.012 5 =
   a. 4
   b. 0.4
   c. 0.25

5. 1/6 × 5/8 =

   a. $\dfrac{5}{40}$ b. $\dfrac{5}{48}$ c. $\dfrac{8}{30}$

6. 5/24 ÷ 1/3 =

   a. $\dfrac{5}{6}$ b. $\dfrac{5}{72}$ c. $\dfrac{15}{24}$

7. Which of the following abbreviations means that a drug is to be administered at bedtime?
   a. ac
   b. pc
   c. hs

8. How many grams are equivalent to 105 mg?
   a. 105 000
   b. 0.105
   c. 1.05

9. The IV order states: infuse 3 000 mL/day. Using a set with a drop factor of 10 drops/mL, calculate rate of flow in mL/hour.
   a. 125
   b. 1 250
   c. 21

10. How many mL of solution are in the syringe below?
    a. 22 mL
    b. 0.22 mL
    c. 2.2 mL

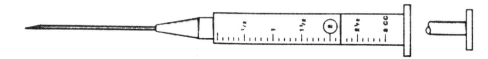

11. The drug is available in 250 mg tablets. How many tablets are required for a dose of 0.5 g?
    a. 0.5
    b. 2
    c. 5

12. The vial label states: regular insulin 100 units/mL. How many units in 0.34 mL?
    a. 34
    b. 0.34
    c. 3.4

13. The order is for 750 000 units of penicillin G; the label states that there are 300 000 units/mL. How many mL are required?
    a. 2.5 mL
    b. 0.4 mL
    c. 0.25 mL

14. The label on the penicillin states 1 000 000 units/mL. How mnay units are found in 2.3 mL?
    a. 2 300 000
    b. 230 000
    c. 23 000 000

15. The order is for 12.5 mg. The medication is supplied as a syrup with the concentration of 25 mg/5 mL. How many tsp are required?
    a. 2.5
    b. 2
    c. 0.5

16. Which of the following tablets provides the largest amount of medication?
    a. 0.1 mg
    b. 0.05 mg
    c. 0.15 mg

17. The order: 45 mg IM stat. Available: a 2 mL ampule with solution concentration of 50 mg/mL. How many mL should be given?
    a. 1.8
    b. 0.9
    c. 1.1

18. Ordered: Theo-Dur 900 mg PO in 3 divided doses. Available: 0.3 g tablets. What is the amount to administer for each dose?
    a. 3 tab
    b. 1 tab
    c. 9 tab

19. A 1 L bag of IV solution is infusing at 75 mL/hour and has been running for 3 hours and 30 minutes. How much solution should have been infused?
    a. 262.5
    b. 225
    c. 737.5

20. Two hundred milligrams of a drug is added to 500 mL of IV solution. What is the concentration in mcg/mL?
    a. 400
    b. 0.4
    c. 2.5

ANSWER GUIDE

NOTE: This Answer Guide is provided for you to check your answers to all exercises, additional practice activities, and posttests. For those questions requiring basic arithmetic skills, only the answer is provided. For more complex skills, an example showing the process used to obtain the answer is provided. These examples are intended to assist you in analyzing any mistakes. To prevent a cumbersome answer guide, however, not all calculations will be shown.

Module 1 Pretest

Arithmetic of Whole Numbers

1. 1 223
2. 2 517
3. 814
4. 594
5. 475
6. 1 354
7. 53
8. 789
9. 51 684
10. 8 385
11. 890 415
12. 2 189 094
13. 5
14. 8
15. 5

7. $2\frac{3}{4}$

8. $7\frac{7}{24}$

9. $\frac{7}{16}$

10. $\frac{1}{4}$

11. $\frac{7}{24}$

12. $\frac{1}{24}$

13. $\frac{47}{72}$

14. $\frac{13}{20}$

15. $2\frac{9}{16}$

16. $2\frac{15}{16}$

17. $28\frac{31}{56}$

18. $1\frac{5}{12}$

19. $7\frac{29}{64}$

20. $8\frac{1}{3}$

Arithmetic of Fractions

1. $\frac{34}{39}$

2. $\frac{101}{112}$

3. $\frac{23}{30}$

4. $1\frac{5}{12}$

5. $3\frac{13}{20}$

6. $1\frac{7}{30}$

21. $\dfrac{1}{2}$

22. $14\dfrac{5}{8}$

23. $4\dfrac{4}{5}$

24. $31\dfrac{1}{2}$

25. $1\dfrac{11}{24}$

26. $\dfrac{3}{4}$

27. $9\dfrac{3}{4}$

28. $\dfrac{50}{63}$

29. $\dfrac{8}{9}$

30. 3

31. $101\dfrac{1}{3}$

32. $\dfrac{3}{16}$

33. $3\dfrac{3}{5}$

34. $7\dfrac{6}{11}$

35. $8\dfrac{1}{6}$

36. $3\dfrac{25}{34}$

37. $4\dfrac{7}{8}$

38. $10\dfrac{5}{12}$

39. 4

40. 30

41. 40

42. 24

43. $\dfrac{7}{8}$

44. $\dfrac{1}{4}$

45. $\dfrac{2}{3}$

46. $\dfrac{3}{7}$

47. $\dfrac{5}{8}$

48. $\dfrac{1}{15}$

49. proper

50. improper

51. mixed

52. proper

53. proper

54. proper

55. mixed

56. improper

57. 3; complete fraction is: $\dfrac{3}{6}$

58. 60; complete fraction is: $\dfrac{9}{60}$

59. 21; complete fraction is: $\dfrac{21}{27}$

60. 70; complete fraction is: $\dfrac{49}{70}$

61. 30; complete fraction is: $\dfrac{6}{30}$

62. no

63. yes

64. $\dfrac{49}{8}$

65. $\dfrac{79}{10}$

66. $\dfrac{11}{2}$

67. 0.25

68. 1

69. 0.12

70. 0.5

Arithmetic of Decimal Numbers

1. 0.5
2. 3.4
3. 7.1
4. 1.2
5. 9.2
6. 12.46
7. 6.09
8. 34.01
9. 4.91
10. 2.547
11. 126.034 2
12. 6.27
13. 3.732
14. 6.3
15. 3.3
16. 4.52
17. 0.05
18. 8
19. 80
20. 800
21. 0.001
22. 0.5
23. 66.7
24. 2.2
25. 44.5
26. 0.8
27. 0.5
28. 0.3
29. 0.8
30. 0.6
31. 1.9
32. $\frac{3}{5}$
33. $\frac{57}{100}$
34. $1\frac{1}{4}$
35. $\frac{1}{100}$
36. 1.01, 0.1, 0.01, 0.001
37. $\frac{1}{4}$
38. 0.25
39. 0.83
40. 83%
41. $\frac{1}{1\,000}$
42. 0.1%
43. 1.75
44. 175%
45. 1.901, 1.991, 10.01, 10.1

Module 1 Posttest

1. 111
2. 377
3. 18
4. 282
5. 3 479
6. 60 564
7. 6
8. 7.3
9. $\frac{25}{28}$
10. $1\frac{21}{40}$
11. $\frac{13}{14}$
12. $14\frac{7}{12}$
13. $\frac{37}{60}$
14. $1\frac{7}{8}$
15. $1\frac{11}{21}$
16. $\frac{31}{32}$
17. $\frac{17}{36}$
18. $2\frac{1}{3}$
19. $1\frac{1}{5}$

20. $20\dfrac{1}{16}$

21. $\dfrac{5}{24}$

22. $\dfrac{43}{120}$

23. $\dfrac{5}{28}$

24. $\dfrac{17}{144}$

25. $\dfrac{6}{63}$

26. $\dfrac{3}{5}$

27. 75

28. $7\dfrac{2}{3}$

29. 3

30. 78

31. $1\dfrac{1}{4}$

32. $\dfrac{3}{16}$

33. $\dfrac{3}{4}$

34. $9\dfrac{3}{4}$

35. $\dfrac{9}{10}$

36. $\dfrac{5}{12}$

37. $\dfrac{50}{63}$

38. $13\dfrac{1}{3}$

39. $133\dfrac{1}{3}$

40. 22

41. $\dfrac{38}{3}$

42. $\dfrac{14}{4}$

43. $4\dfrac{1}{5}$

44. $4\dfrac{2}{9}$

45. $2\dfrac{3}{4}$

46. $12\dfrac{5}{7}$

47. $16\dfrac{11}{12}$

48. $3\dfrac{1}{3}$

49. 72

50. 48

51. 72

52. 42

53. $\dfrac{4}{9}$

54. $\dfrac{5}{9}$

55. $\dfrac{5}{6}$

56. 3

57. $\dfrac{8}{9}$

58. $\dfrac{14}{11}$

59. $1\dfrac{2}{3}$

60. 49; complete fraction is: $\dfrac{35}{49}$

61. 70; complete fraction is: $\dfrac{28}{70}$

62. 60; complete fraction is: $\dfrac{60}{108}$

63. 30; complete fraction is: $\dfrac{30}{200}$

64. 44; complete fraction is: $\dfrac{32}{44}$

65. 4.15
66. 1.77
67. 1.26
68. 1.32
69. 2.3
70. 1.9
71. 1.2
72. 2.4
73. 10.626
74. 0.303
75. 4.25
76. 101
77. 180
78. 0.125
79. 2
80. 3
81. 4.2
82. 1.8
83. 1.3
84. 2.3
85. 1.89
86. 1.97
87. 10.64
88. 0.36
89. 0.67
90. 67%

91. $\dfrac{22}{25}$

92. 88%

93. $\dfrac{37}{100}$

94. 0.37
95. 3.8
96. 380%

97. $1\dfrac{1}{5}$

98. 120%

99. $\dfrac{3}{1\,000}$

100. 0.003

Module 2

Exercise 2.1

1. 2:18 (or 1:9)
2. 18:20 (or 9:10)
3. 325 units:1 tab
4. 25 units:1 tsp
5. 12:48 (or 1:4)

Exercise 2.2

1. $\dfrac{1}{25}$

2. 0.04
3. 4%
4. 1:10
5. 0.1
6. 10%
7. 7:9

8. $\dfrac{7}{9}$

9. 78%
10. 1:3

11. $\dfrac{1}{3}$

12. 0.333
13. 50:1
14. 50
15. 5 000%

Exercise 2.3

Example solution:

1. Solve by multiplying means and extremes: Solve by using cross product:

    $3 \times x = 2 \times 12$

    $3x = 24$

    $x = \dfrac{24}{3} = 8$

    validate 3 x 8 = 2 × 12

    $\dfrac{2}{3} = \dfrac{x}{12}$

    $3 \times x = 2 \times 12$

    $3x = 24$

    $x = 8$

    validate: $3 \times 8 = 2 \times 12$

2. 25
3. 21
4. 2
5. 1.5
6. 4
7. 0.35
8. 0.5
9. 0.25
10. 1
11. 4
12. 1 080
13. 1
14. 0.5 Example solution when ratio is expressed as fraction: first convert fraction to a

    decimal number: $\dfrac{1}{4} = 0.25$; then solve: 0.25: x = 6.12: 6x = 0.25 × 12

    $x = \dfrac{3}{6} = 0.5$

15. 0.6

16. 16 scoops   6 (cups): 4 (scoops) = 24 (cups): x (scoops)
    $6x = 4 \times 24 = 96$

    $x = \dfrac{96}{6} = 16$

    Validation
    6:4 = 24:16
    96 = 96

17. 4 cups   express $1\dfrac{1}{2}$ as 1.5

    1 (c milk):1.5(c mix) = x(c milk): 6(c mix)
    1.5 x = 6
    x = 4
    Validation
    1:1.5 = 4:6
    6 = 6

18. 15 gum

$1 \text{ (gum)}: 3 \text{ (mints)} = x \text{ (gum)}:45 \text{ (mints)}$
$3x = 45: x = 15$
$1:3 = 15:45; 3 \times 15 = 1 \times 45; 45 = 45$

19. 42 hot dogs

$22 \text{ (children)}: 33 \text{ (hot dogs)} = 28 \text{ children}: x \text{ (hotdogs)}$

$22x = 33 \times 28; x = \dfrac{924}{22} = 42$

$22:33 = 28:42; 33 \times 28 = 22 \times 42; 924 = 924$

20. 8 cups

$1 \text{ (lime)}: 3 \text{ (apple)} = x \text{ (lime)}: 24 \text{ (apple)}$

$3x = 24; x = \dfrac{24}{3} = 8$

$1:3 = 8:24; 3 \times 8 = 24$

Exercise 2.4

1. 45
2. 12
3. 25
4. 4
5. 4
6. 3
7. $\dfrac{1}{100}$
8. 0.01
9. 1%
10. $\dfrac{1}{5}$
11. 0.2
12. 20%
13. $\dfrac{1}{250}$
14. 0.004
15. 0.4%
16. 0.5
17. 165
18. 2 000
19. 12.5
20. 7:5
21. 5:1
22. 17:3
23. 1.5
24. relationship that exists between two quantities
25. expression of two equal or equivalent ratios
26. 15

27. 15
28. 36
29. 1.5
30. 20

Module 2 Posttest

1. 9
2. 8
3. 10
4. 23:39
5. 3:17
6. 7
7. relationship that exists between two quantities
8. expression of two equal or equivalent ratios
9. 1:10
10. no
11. 9:1 000
12. $\dfrac{1}{1}$
13. 1
14. 100%
15. 2:3
16. 0.67
17. 67%
18. 1:1 000
19. $\dfrac{1}{1\,000}$
20. 0.1%
21. $\dfrac{3}{250}$

22. $\dfrac{4}{125}$

23. $\dfrac{1}{8}$

24. $\dfrac{2}{5}$

25. 1 (red):8 (green) = 12 (red):x (green)
26. 1x = 8 × 12; x = 96
27. 1:8 = 12:96; 8 × 12 = 1 × 96; 96=96
28. 1.5 (tbsp):3 (cups) = x (tbsp):8 (cups)

29. $3x = 1.5 \times 8; x = \dfrac{12}{3} = 4$

30. 1.5:3 = 4:8; 12 = 12

Module 3

Exercise 3.1

1. K
2. d
3. c
4. m
5. mc OR μ
6. 1 000
7. 0.000 000 001
8. 0.000 000 000 001
9. 0.001
10. 0.000 001
11. 0.01
12. 100
13. kilo, hecto, deci, centi, milli, micro, nano, pico

Exercise 3.2

1. m
2. 10 kg
3. 0.5 mL
4. L
5. 1 000 mL
6. 0.5 L
7. 1 050 mg
8. mL
9. 51 517
10. true

Exercise 3.3

1. 1 000
2. 1 000
3. 100
4. 1
5. 1 000 000
6. 0.25
7. 500
8. 200
9. 1 000
10. 0.001
11. 0.3
12. 0.8
13. 1.5
14. 750

Exercise 3.4

1. 79.545
2. 79.5
3. 80
4. 55.118
5. 4 ft and 7 in
6. 5
7. 30
8. 160.02
9. 2
10. 750
11. 59.4
12. 15
13. 76.2
14. 9.46
15. 167.6
16. 60
17. 67.7
18. 1 000
19. 60.6
20. 8

Exercise 3.5

1. 103.6
2. 40.1
3. 96.8
4. 38
5. 11.1
6. 75.2

7. −22.2
8. 10.4
9. −11.1

Exercise 3.6

1. 10 000
2. 0.05
3. 250
4. 1 250
5. 1 000
6. 2 000
7. 0.35
8. 150
9. 700 000
10. 102
11. 10
12. 77
13. 65
14. 66.66
15. 17
16. 960
17. 2 160
18. 61
19. 3
20. 31

Exercise 3.7

1. metre, m
2. kilogram, kg
3. mole, mol
4. 0.1
5. 0.01
6. 0.001
7. 0.000 000 001
8. 0.000 001
9. 1 000
10. 1 000
11. 1 000
12. 0.01
13. 1 000
14. 0.001
15. 0.25
16. 0.04
17. 0.2
18. 300
19. 100
20. 2.5
21. 600

22. 60
23. 5
24. 6.6
25. 182.88

Module 3 Posttest

1. 2 000
2. 0.25
3. 2
4. 6 000
5. 7 000
6. 5
7. 0.001 25
8. 3
9. 2 500
10. 500
11. 1.456
12. 0.000 5
13. 1 000
14. 170
15. 1.79
16. 500
17. 0.25
18. 1 340
19. 10 000 000
20. 79 000 000
21. 0.01
22. 0.001
23. 0.000 001
24. 1 000
25. 0.1
26. 10
27. 180
28. 3.64
29. 22
30. 31.5
31. 20
32. 185.4
33. 101.48
34. 55
35. 0.48
36. 94.5
37. 23.9
38. 45
39. 1 500
40. 98.6

Module 4

Exercise 4.1

1. intramuscularly every 3 to 4 hours as necessary
2. by mouth every 4 hours
3. by mouth immediately and every 4 hours
4. intravenously 4 times a day
5. elixir 100 milligrams at bedtime
6. patient's name, drug, dosage, route, time/frequency of administration, date, and physician's signature.
7. freely, as needed
8. drop
9. sublingual
10. suppository
11. after meals (1/2 hour after meals)
12. tablet
13. twice a day
14. at bedtime
15. ointment
16. milligram
17. microgram
18. subcutaneous
19. extract
20. before meals (1/2 hour before meals)
21. intramuscular
22. as much as required
23. with
24. immediately

Exercise 4.2

1. solution
2. solute
3. solvent
4. penicillin G potassium
5. sterile water
6. true
7. b
8. a
9. g
10. mL
11. mL
12. mL
13. w/v (weight/volume)
14. v/v (volume/volume)
15. water, normal saline, alcohol

Exercise 4.3

1. tablet
2. 325 mg
3. acetaminophen
4. Colace
5. docusate sodium
6. 1 – 3 tablespoons or 5 – 15 mL
7. liquid
8. 20 mg/5 mL or 4 mg/mL
9. 8 fl oz = 8 × 30 = 240 mL
10. 24 days (2 tsp = 10 mL)

Exercise 4.4

1. intramuscularly every 4 hours as necessary
2. subcutaneous immediately
3. by mouth before meals (1/2 hour before meals) 3 times a day
4. by mouth 1 hour after meals 3 times a day
5. by mouth at bedtime
6. tablet
7. liquid
8. 5 mg/tablet
9. 10 mg/mL
10. dose
11. route
12. false
13. E
14. G
15. F
16. C
17. H
18. I
19. B
20. A
21. D
22. J
23. 75 mL; 33 mL; 11.5 mL
24. 20 million units
25. 500 000 U/mL
26. penicillin G potassium
27. Pfizerpen
28. intravenous
29. 6 – 40 million units
30. twenty-second day (of the month)
31. substance dissolved in a solution

32. homogenous mixture that contains one or more dissolved substances in a solution
33. liquid in which another substance is dissolved
34. determined by amount of solute dissolved in a given amount of solvent

Exercise 4.5

1. solution
2. 10 mg/mL
3. tablet
4. 125 mg per tab
5. tablet
6. 300 mg per tab
7. liquid/solution
8. 50 mg per mL
9. liquid/solution
10. 5 mg per mL
11. liquid/solution
12. 1 mg per mL
13. liquid/solution
14. 2.5 mg per mL
15. liquid/solution
16. 1 000 IU. per mL
17. liquid/solution
18. 25 mg per mL
19. liquid/solution
20. 2.67 mEq per mL
21. 800 (for answers 21 – 30; recall 1 mg = 1 000 mcg)
22. 0.8
23. 600
24. 0.6
25. 400
26. 0.4
27. 320
28. 0.32
29. 200
30. 0.2

Exercise 4.6

1. acetaminophen
2. tablets
3. 325 mg per tab
4. acetaminophen
5. liquid/solution
6. 32 mg/mL
7. indocin
8. indomethacin
9. capsule
10. 75 mg per capsule
11. 60
12. Indocin
13. indomethacin
14. capsule
15. 25 mg per capsule
16. 100
17. 1%
18. 1 part per 100
19. 10 mg
20. 50 mg
21. 5 mL
22. 20 000 IU (20 × 1 000)
23. 1 000 IU per mL; heparin sodium
24. 20 mL
25. 10 000 IU per mL
26. 5 mL
27. 100 IU per mL
28. 1 mL
29. 10 000 IU per mL — Label B
30. intravenous or subcutaneous

Module 4 Posttest

Part I

Crossword

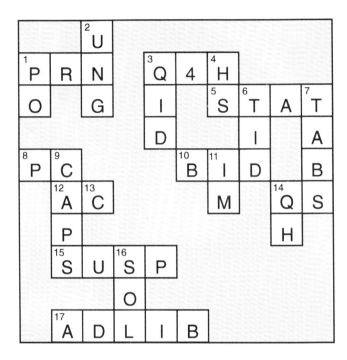

Part II

1. powder
2. intravenous
3. 250 mg to 1 gram
4. every 6 to 12 hours
5. sterile water for injection
6. 96 mL
7. 200 mg per mL
8. 10 grams

Part III

1. Give digoxin 250 micrograms by mouth daily
2. Give Demerol 75 milligrams intramuscularly every 3 to 4 hours as necessary
3. Nitro spray sublingually as necessary
4. Nifedipine 20 milligram tablets by mouth 2 times a day
5. Nitroglycerin 0.3 milligram tablets sublingually as necessary at bedside
6. Procainamide slow (or sustained) release tablets, 750 milligrams by mouth 3 times a day
7. Glycerin suppository per rectum as necessary.
8. Salbutamol inhaler, 100 micrograms per dose, 2 puffs every 4 to 6 hours

Part IV

1. heparin sodium (the drug is the solute)
2. 25 000 international units in each millilitre
3. benzyl alcohol 1%; methylparahydroxybenzoate 0.1%; and propylparahydroxybenzoate 0.02%

Exercise 5.1

1. Sample calculations

Method A: Proportion - extremes/means

$$300:1 = 450:x$$

$$300x = 450$$

$x = 1.5$ Give 1.5 (or $1\frac{1}{2}$) tabs

Validation:

$$300:1 = 450:1.5$$

$$450 = 450$$

Method B: Proportion - cross product

$$\frac{300}{1} = \frac{450}{x}$$

$$300x = 450$$

$x = 1.5$ Give 1.5 (or $1\frac{1}{2}$) tabs

Validation:

$$\frac{300}{1} = \frac{450}{1.5}$$

$$450 = 450$$

Method C: dose/supply

$$\frac{dose}{supply} = \frac{450}{300} = 1.5 \text{ (or } 1\frac{1}{2}\text{) tabs}$$

Note — to validate use either Method A or Method B. You cannot validate if you use the formula.

2.	2 tabs	3.	0.5 tab	4.	1.5 tabs
5.	2 tabs	6.	1 (20 mg) and 2 (5 mg) tabs	7.	0.5 tab
8.	2 tabs	9.	0.5 tab	10.	2 tabs

Exercise 5.2

1.   Sample Calculation
      Express both doses in mg:
      0.015 g = x mg (recall 1 g = 1 000 mg): 0.015 g = 15 mg

Method A

5 mg:1 tab = 15 mg:x tab

5x = 15
x = 3 Give 3 tabs
Validation:

5:1 = 15 : 3

15 = 15

Method B

$$\frac{5}{1} = \frac{15}{x}$$
5x = 15
x = 3
Validation

$$\frac{5}{1} = \frac{15}{3}$$
15 = 15

Method C

$$\frac{dose}{supply} = \frac{15\ mg}{5\ mg} = 3\ tabs$$

Note — to validate use either Method A or Method B. You cannot validate if you use the formula.

2.	3 tabs	3.	2 tabs	4.	4 tabs		
5.	2 tabs	6.	2 caps	7.	3 tabs		
8.	1 tab	9.	168 caps	10.	1 tab (125 mcg)		

Exercise 5.3

1.   (a) 15 mg tab
      (b) give 1 tab
2.   (a) 10 mg tab
      (b) give 1 tab
3.   (a) 100 mg cap
      (b) give 2 caps
4.   (a) 15 mg tab
      (b) give 1 tab in am
      (c) 30 mg tab
      (d) give 1 tab at hs
5.   (a) 0.25 mg tab
      (b) give 1 tab
6.   250 mcg (or µg)
7.   1 (15 mg) tab
      (b) 1 (10 mg) tab
      (c) need 1 (15 mg tab) × 3/day × 4 days = 12 (15 mg) tablets and 1 (10 mg tab) × 3/day ×
      3 days = 9 (10 mg) tablets

8. 300 mg
9. (a) 1 (30 mg tab) twice a day
   (b) 1 (30 mg tab) with 1 (15 mg tab) at hs.
   (c) Total daily dose: $(30 \times 2) + 45 = 105$ mg

Exercise 5.4

1. a. 2 caps
   b. 4 caps
2. a. 3 tabs
   b. 3 tabs
3. a. 2 tabs
   b. 8 tabs
4. a. 3 tabs
   b. 3 tabs
5. a. 1.5 tabs
   b. 4.5 tabs
6. a. 1 tab
   b. 1 tab
7. a. 2 tabs
   b. 8 tabs
8. a. 2 tabs
   b. 8 tabs
9. a. 2 tabs
   b. 4 tabs
10. a. 2 tabs
    b. 8 tabs

Exercise 5.5

1. 25
2. 200
3. 500
4. 120 (4 × 30 mL)
5. 237 (or 240) (NOTE)
6. 5 mL
7. 1 tsp
8. 10 mL
9. 4 mL
10. 1 tsp
11. 7.5 mL
12. 2.5 mL
13. 4 mL
14. 1 tsp
15. 10 mL
16. 48 doses (approx 5 mL each)
17. 6 doses each dose 20 mL
18. 40 doses each dose 5 mL
19. 2 doses each dose 10 mL
20. approx 33 doses each dose 15 mL

NOTE: 1 fluid ounce = 30 mL, therefore 8 fl oz should = 240 mL but manufacturer is not using SI system.

Exercise 5.6

1. Give 3 tabs

   Convert:
   0.3 g = x mg = 300 mg
   100 mg:1 tab = 300 mg:x tab
   100x = 300
   x = 3

   Validate: Proportion: extremes × means

   100 mg:1 tab = 300 mg:3 tabs

   300 = 300

2. Give 2 tabs

   $$\frac{dose}{supply} = x \text{ tab}$$

   $$\frac{2.5 \text{ mg}}{1 \text{ tab}} = \frac{5 \text{ mg}}{x \text{ tab}}$$

   2.5x = 5
   x = 2

   Validate: Proportion: extremes × means

   2.5 mg:1 tab = 5 mg:2 tab

   5 = 5

3. Give 2.5 tabs   Convert: 2 500 mg = 2.5 g   Proportion: extremes × means

$$\frac{1\ g}{1\ tab} = \frac{2.5\ g}{x\ tab}$$

1 g:1 tab = 2.5 g:2.5 tabs

325x = 650
x = 2.5   2.5 = 2.5

4. Give 10 mL   15 mg:5 mL = 30 mg:x mL   Proportion: extremes × means
                    15x = 150
                    x = 10   15 mg:5 mL = 30 mg:10 mL

                                                 15 x 10 = 5 x 30
                                                 150 = 150

5. Give 0.5 tab $\dfrac{0.25\ mg}{1\ tab} = \dfrac{0.125\ mg}{x\ tab}$ Proportion: extremes × means

                    0.25x = 0.125   0.25 mg:1 tab = 0.125 mg:0.5 tabs

                    $x = \dfrac{0.125}{0.25} = \dfrac{12.5}{25} = 0.5$ 0.125 = 0.125

Additional Practice

1. | **Generic** | **Trade** |
    |---|---|
    | levothyroxine sodium | Eltroxin |
    | levothyroxine sodium | Synthroid |
    | digoxin | Lanoxin |
    | furosemide | Lasix |
    | indapamide | Lozide |
    | omeprazole | Losec |

2. | **Drug** | **Available strengths** |
    |---|---|
    | Lanoxin | 0.25 mg; 0.125 mg; 0.0625 mg |
    | Lasix | 20 mg; 40 mg; 80 mg |
    | Synthroid | 0.05 mg; 0.1 mg; 0.15 mg; 0.025 mg |
    | Eltroxin | 300 mcg; 50 mcg |

3. **Today's doses**
    give 1 tab of 80 mg Lasix
    give 1 tab of 0.25 mg and 1 tab of 0.125 mg digoxin or give 3 tabs of 0.125 mg strength
    give 3 tabs of 0.025 mg Synthroid

4. **Tomorrow's doses**
    give 1 tab of 40 mg Lasix
    give 1 tab of 0.25 mg digoxin
    give 3 tabs of 0.025 mg Synthroid

5. 0.15 mg; 0.1 mg; 0.05 mg; 0.025 mg. (NOTE: if unsure about the relative size of decimal numbers write in a column and compare:
    0.150
    0.100
    0.050
    0.025

6. day 1: 3 (20 mg) tabs in am
    day 2: 4 (20 mg) tabs in am
    day 3: 3 (20 mg) tabs in am (NOTE: order for 60 mg in am and 60 mg in pm)

7. give 1 (2.5 mg) tab

8. Eltroxin 300 mcg, 1 tab is the most accurate and simplest to administer; the alternate choice is 3 (0.1 mg) tabs of Synthroid but less desirable to give 3 tablets.

9. 1. Synthroid: 1 (0.05 mg) tab
    2. Synthroid: 2 (0.025 mg) tabs
    3. Eltroxin: 1 (50 mcg) tab
    4. Use either Synthroid 0.05 mg tab or Eltroxin 50 mcg tab

10. 0.4375 mg

11. 0.25 mg = 250 mcg
    0.125 mg = 125 mcg
    0.0625 mg = 62.5 mcg
    (NOTE: with this conversion, the comparative strengths are more obvious).

12. give 2 (40 mg) tabs; give 4 (20 mg) tabs; give 2 (20 mg) plus 1 (40 mg) tab.

13. give 1 tab (0.1 mg) Synthroid

14. give 1 tab (0.125 mg) digoxin

15. give 1 tab (20 mg) omeprazole (Losec)

Module 5 Posttest

Score 1 point for correct answer in each column (i.e., 1 for correct unit, 1 for correct calculation and answer 1 for validation).

ANSWER correct unit	CALCULATION	VALIDATION different methods are shown **always check that units are consistent across the equation**
1. Give 3 tabs	Convert: 0.3 g = x mg = 300 mg 100 mg:1 tab = 300 mg:x tab 100x = 300 x = 3	Proportion: extremes × means 100 mg:1 tab = 300 mg:3 tabs 300 = 300

2. Give 0.5 tab

$$\frac{2.5\text{ mg}}{1\text{ tab}} = \frac{1.25\text{ mg}}{x\text{ tab}}$$

Proportion: cross product

$$2.5x = 1.25$$

$$\frac{2.5\text{ mg}}{1\text{ tab}} = \frac{1.25\text{ mg}}{0.5\text{ tab}}$$

$$x = 0.5$$

$$1.25 = 1.25$$

3. If today's date is:
    even – 1 tab
    odd – 2 tabs

$$\frac{\text{dose}}{\text{supply}} = x\text{ tab}$$

Even days: $\dfrac{2.5\text{ mg}}{2.5\text{ mg}} = 1$ tab

Odd days: $\dfrac{5\text{ mg}}{2.5\text{ mg}} = 2$ tabs

Validation: note, if you use the formula, you must use proportion to validate
2.5 mg:1 tab = 5 mg:2 tab
5 = 5

4. Give 2 tabs

Convert: 0.65 g - 650 mg
325 mg:1 tab = 650 mg:x tab
$325x = 650$
$x = 2$

Proportion: extremes × means

325 mg:1 tab = 650 mg:2 tabs

$650 = 650$

5. Give 2 tab

$$\frac{0.4\text{ mg}}{1\text{ tab}} = \frac{0.8\text{ mg}}{x\text{ tab}}$$

Proportion: cross product

$$0.4x = 0.8$$

$$\frac{0.4\text{ mg}}{1\text{ tab}} = \frac{0.8\text{ mg}}{2\text{ tabs}}$$

$$x = 2$$

$$2 = 2$$

6. 2-week supply

= 14 tabs (1 per day)

Convert 125 mcg = 0.125 mg

$$\frac{\text{dose}}{\text{supply}} = \frac{0.125}{0.125} = 1\text{ tab}$$

1 tab x 14 days = 14 tabs

Note: to validate chose one of the proportion methods.

7. Give 2.5 tabs

Convert: 2 500 mg = 2.5 g
1 g:1 tab = 2.5 g:x tab
$x = 2.5$

Proportion: extremes × means

1 g:1 tab = 2.5 g:2.5 tabs

$2.5 = 2.5$

8. Give 1.5 tab

$$\frac{50\text{ mg}}{1\text{ tab}} = \frac{75\text{ mg}}{x\text{ tab}}$$

Proportion: cross product

$$50x = 75$$

$$\frac{50\text{ mg}}{1\text{ tab}} = \frac{75\text{ mg}}{1.5\text{ tab}}$$

$$x = 2.5$$

$$75 = 75$$

9. Actual dose is 36 mg

15 mg:5 mL = x mg:12 mL
5x = 180
x = 36

Proportion: extremes × means

15 mg:5 mL = 36 mg:12 mL

$15 \times 12 = 5 \times 36$
180 = 180

10. Give 10 mL

25 mg:5 mL = 500 mg:x mL

250x = 2 500

x = 10

Proportion: cross product

$\dfrac{250 \text{ mg}}{5 \text{ mL}} = \dfrac{500 \text{ mg}}{10 \text{ mL}}$

750 = 750

11. Give 4mL (round to whole number)

$\dfrac{200 \text{ mg}}{5 \text{ mL}} = \dfrac{150 \text{ mg}}{x \text{ mL}}$

200x = 750

x = 3.75

Proportion: cross product

$\dfrac{200 \text{ mg}}{5 \text{ mL}} = \dfrac{150 \text{ mg}}{3.75 \text{ mL}}$

750 = 750

12. Received 200 mg

Convert 1 tsp = 5 mL
Read label: 200 mg per 5 mL

To validate: read label again — in the clinical setting you should read the label 3 times!

13. Give 2 mL (round to whole number)

200 mg:5 mL = 75 mg:x mL

200x = 375

x = 1.875

Proportion: cross product

$\dfrac{200 \text{ mg}}{5 \text{ mL}} = \dfrac{75 \text{ mg}}{1.875 \text{ mL}}$

375 = 375

14. Give 0.5 tab

0.25 mg:1 tab = 0.125 mg:x tab
0.25x = 0.125
x = 0.5

Proportion: extremes × means

0.25 mg:1 tab = 0.125 mg:0.5 tabs

0.125 = 0.125

15. Give 4 mL

$\dfrac{125 \text{ mg}}{5 \text{ mL}} = \dfrac{100 \text{ mg}}{x \text{ mL}}$

125x = 500

x = 4

Proportion: extremes × means

$\dfrac{125 \text{ mg}}{5 \text{ mL}} = \dfrac{100 \text{ mg}}{4 \text{ mL}}$

500 = 500

16. Each mg = 1 600 units

$\dfrac{125 \text{ mg}}{200\,000 \text{ units}} = \dfrac{1 \text{ mg}}{x \text{ units}}$

125x = 200 000

x = 1 600

Proportion: cross product

$\dfrac{125 \text{ mg}}{200\,000 \text{ units}} = \dfrac{1 \text{ mg}}{1\,600 \text{ units}}$

200 000 = 200 000

17. Give 3 mL
(round to
whole number)

$$\frac{200\ 000\ \text{units}}{5\ \text{mL}} = \frac{125\ 000\ \text{units}}{x\ \text{mL}}$$ Proportion: cross product

$200\ 000x = 625\ 000$

$x = 3.1$

$$\frac{200\ 000\ \text{units}}{5\ \text{mL}} = \frac{125\ 000\ \text{units}}{3.125\ \text{mL}}$$

$625\ 000 = 625\ 000$

18. 375 mcg in
1.5 tabs

250 mcg:1 tab = x mcg:1.5 tab   Proportion: extremes × means

$0.25x = 0.125$

$x = 375$

250 mcg:1 tab = 375 mcg:1.5 tabs

$375 = 375$

19. 2 500 mg
(or 4 million
units)

$$\frac{125\ \text{mg}}{5\ \text{mL}} = \frac{x\ \text{mg}}{100\ \text{mL}}$$ Proportion: cross multiplication

$5x = 12\ 500$

$x = 2\ 500$

$$\frac{125\ \text{mg}}{5\ \text{mL}} = \frac{2\ 500\ \text{mg}}{100\ \text{mL}}$$

$12\ 500 = 12\ 500$

20. 40 000 units

$$\frac{200\ 000\ \text{units}}{5\ \text{mL}} = \frac{x\ \text{units}}{1\ \text{mL}}$$ Proportion: cross multiplication

$5x = 200\ 000$
$x = 40\ 000$

200 000 units:5 mL = 40 000 units:1 mL
$200\ 000 = 200\ 000$

Module 6

Exercise 6.1

1   (a) 1 mL (or cc)   (b) 0.65 mL

2   (a) 2.5 mL or $(2\frac{1}{2})$ mL   (b) 2.1 mL

3   (a) 3 mL (or cc)   (b) 1.8 mL

4   (a) 1 mL (or cc)   (b) 0.72 mL

5   (a) 2.5 mL or $(2\frac{1}{2})$ mL   (b) 1.5 mL

Exercise 6.2

1.   Sample calculation using proportion method
      10 000 units:1 mL = 7 500 units:x mL
      10 000x = 7 500
      x = 7 500 / 10 000 = 0.75
      Give 0.75 mL

2.   Known ratio: 50 mg:1 mL
      Unknown ratio: x mg:1.5 mL
      Solve: 50:1 = x:1.5
      x = 75 mg

3. $\dfrac{250}{1} = \dfrac{400}{x}$
      250 x = 400
      x = 1.6 (Give 1.6 mL)
      Validate: 250:1 = 400:1.6 (400 = 400)

4.   1.5 mL

5.   0.8 mL

6.   Convert: 200 mg = x units (200 × 1 600 = 320 000)
      Solve: 400 000:1 = 320 000:x
      x = 0.8 (Give 0.8 mL)
      Validate: 400 000:1 = 32 000:0.8 (320 000 = 320 000)

7.   0.5 mL

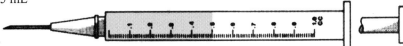

8.   0.8 mL

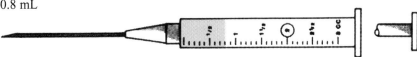

9.   0.6 mL

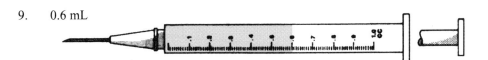

10.   1.5 mL

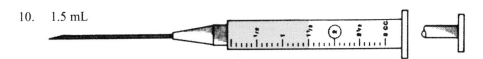

Exercise 6.3

1. 0.46 mL
2. 2.4 mL
3. 1.2 mL
4. 0.78 mL
5. 32 units (or 0.32 mL)
6. 0.85 mL
7. 54 units (or 0.54 mL)
8. 0.13 mL

Exercise 6.6

1. No: 0.25 mL
2. 1 mL not 1 ampule
3. No: 0.5 mL
4. No: 4.3 mL
5. yes

Exercise 6.4

1. 9.3 mL
2. 1.3 mL
3. 3.8 mL
4. 2 mL
5. 1.3 mL
6. 250 000 IU
7. 200 000 IU
8. 350 000 IU
9. 1.8 mL sterile water
10. one hour
11. entire vial or 2 mL (1.8 mL diluent + powder = 2 mL)
12. ampicillin sodium
13. ceftizoxime sodium
14. 3 mL sterile or bacteriostatic water for injection
15. 270 mg/mL
16. 24 h room temp; 48 h refrigerator
17. 1.9 mL
18. 2 mL sterile water for injection
19. 1.1 mL
20. 1.8 mL

Exercise 6.5

1. 0.8 mL
2. 0.4 mL
3. 0.7 mL
4. 1.5 mL
5. 0.75 mL
6. 0.6 mL
7. entire vial (volume may be slightly more than 1 mL)
8. 1 g
9. 1.5 mL
10. 2.5 mL

Exercise 6.7

DOSAGE correct unit	CALCULATION	VALIDATION different methods are shown
1. Give 3 mL	250 mg:1.5 mL = 500 mg:x mL 250x = 750 x = 3	Proportion: extremes × means 250:1.5 = 500:3 750 = 750
2. Give 0.8 mL	$\dfrac{10\ mg}{1\ mL} = \dfrac{8\ mg}{x\ mL}$ 10x = 8 x = 0.8	Proportion: cross multiplication $\dfrac{10}{1} = \dfrac{8}{0.8}$ 8 = 8
3. 0.75 mL	$\dfrac{dose\ desired}{dose\ on\ hand} \times vol = amt\ to\ give$ $\dfrac{7.5\ mg}{10\ mg} \times 1\ mL = 0.75\ mL$	validate with proportion
4. 0.75 mL	250 mg:1.5 mL = 125 mg:x mL 250x = 187.5 x = 0.75	Proportion: extremes × means 250:1.5 = 125:0.75 187.5 = 187.5
5. 3 mL	$\dfrac{250\ mg}{1\ mL} = \dfrac{750\ mg}{x\ mL}$ 250x = 750 x = 3	Proportion: cross multiplication $\dfrac{250}{1} = \dfrac{750}{3}$ 750 = 750
6. 6 mg	10 mg:1 mL = x mg:0.6 mL x = 6 mg	10:1 = 6:0.6 6 = 6

7.   2.5 mL
8.   5.7 mL
9.   3.5 mL
10.   approx 330 mg/mL
11.   250 mg/1.5 mL
12.   250 mg/mL
13.   1.5 mL
14.   1.8 mL
15.   375 mg

Additional Practice

Part A

1.   Use product H (morphine 10 mg/mL)
2.   10 mg:1 mL = 8 mg:x mL. Give 0.8 mL
3.   10:1 = 8:0.8
4.

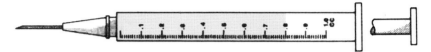

5.   Use C (trade name Ancef)
6.   2.5 mL sterile water
7.   mix and give entire vial contents (approximately 3 mL)
8.   24 h room temp and 96 h in refrigerator
9.   Use A
10.   10 000 units:1 mL = 4 000 units:x mL = 0.4 mL
11.   10 000:1 = 4 000:0.4 (4 000 = 4 000)
12.

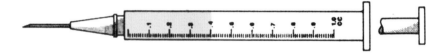

13.   Use F
14.   80 mg:1 mL = 60 mg:x mL Give 0.75 mL
15.   80:1 = 60:0.75 (60 = 60)
16.   shake well immediately before using
17.   not for IV use
18.   use E
19.   Add 5 mL diluent (NOTE. Available vial is 2 g)
20.   330 mg:1 mL = 500 mg:x mL Give 1.5 mL
21.   330:1 = 500:1.5 (500 = 495   NOTE concentration is approximate)
22.   Use G
23.   15 mg:1 mL = 12 mg:x mL Give 0.8 mL
24.   15:1 = 12:0.8 (12 = 12)
25.

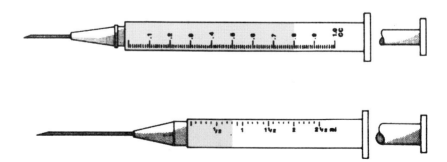

26.   Use D
27.   20 mL
28.   40 mg/mL
29.   40 mg:1 mL = 50 mg:x mL. Give 1.25 mL
30.   40:1 = 50:1.25 (50 = 50)

Part B

1.   sterile water for injection
2.   24 h
3.   72 h
4.   5 g
5.   carbenicillin disodium

6.   IM or IV
7.   add 7 mL water; give 2 mL
8.   add 7 mL water; give 1 mL
9.   0.8 g (or 800 mg)
10.   6 doses ($750 \times 6 = 4\,500$ mg)

Part C

1.   Incorrect. Use Product A not B
2.   Incorrect. Insufficient volume in ampule, use Product G
3.   Incorrect. 2 g vial concentration 330/mL. Give 1.8 mL
4.   Correct
5.   Correct Add 2.5 mL, shake well, withdraw contents of vial (approx. 3 mL)

Case Study

1.   0.6 mL
2.   25 mg:1 mL = 15 mg:0.6 mL
      15 = 15
3.   1 mL
4.   50:1 = 50:1
5.   1 mL

6.   100:1 = 100:1
7.   1 mL
8.   25:1 = 25:1
9.   10 mL PO
10.   160:5 = 325:10

Posttest

1.   100 000 units/mL
2.   2.5 mL
3.   1300 h on 24th day of the month
4.   (a) add 4.6 mL to yield 200 000 unit/mL
      (b) 200 000 units:1 mL = 400 000 units:x mL Give 2 mL
      (c) 200 000:1 = 400 000:2 (400 000 = 400 000)
5.   0.7 mL
6.   1.5 mL
7.   0.75 mL
8.   0.8 mL
9.   1 mL
10.   1.8 mL
11.   6 mg
12.   0.75 mL

13.   3 days room temp, 7 days refrigerator
14.   24 h room temp, 4 days refrigerator
15.   IM or IV
16.   IM or IV
17.   1 g
18.   4 g
19.   Prostaphlin
20.   Staphcillin

Module 7

Exercise 7.1

1. $\dfrac{1\,000\text{ mL}}{(8 \times 60\text{ min})} \times 60\text{ gtts / mL} = 125\text{ gtts / min}$

2. $\dfrac{1\,000\text{ mL}}{(x \times 60\text{ min})} \times 60\text{ gtts / mL} = 50\text{ gtts / min} = 20\text{ hours}$

3. $\dfrac{3\,000\text{ mL}}{(24 \times 60\text{ min})} \times 10\text{ gtts / mL} = 21\text{ gtts / m}$

4. $\dfrac{3\,000\text{ mL}}{(24 \times 60\text{ min})} \times 60\text{ gtts / mL} = 125\text{ gtts / m}$

5. $\dfrac{x\text{ mL}}{(1 \times 60\text{ min})} \times 15\text{ gtts / mL} = 25\text{ gtts / min}$

   $\dfrac{15x}{60} = 25$

   $x = 100\text{ mL per h}$

   Validate:

   $\dfrac{100\text{ mL}}{60\text{ min}} \times 15\text{ gtts / mL} = 25\text{ gtts / min}$

6. $1\,000\text{ mL/8 h}$
7. 125 mL/h

8. $\dfrac{125\text{ mL}}{60\text{ min}} \times 10\text{ gtts / mL} = 21\text{ gtts / min}$

9. $\dfrac{100\text{ mL}}{60\text{ min}} \times 10\text{ gtts / mL} = 17\text{ gtts / min}$

10. $\dfrac{1\,000\text{ mL}}{(6 \times 60\text{ min})} \times 15\text{ gtts / mL} = 42\text{ gtts / min}$

Exercise 7.2

1. 2 mL/min
2. 21 mL/min
3. 83 mL/h
4. 83 gtts/min
5. $2\,000/24 = 83\text{ mL/h}$
6. 21 gtts/min
7. 20 hours

8. $\dfrac{50\text{ mL}}{20\text{ min}} \times 10\text{ gtts / mL} = 25\text{ gtts / min}$

9. $\dfrac{1\,500\text{ mL}}{24 \times 60\text{ min}} \times 20\text{ gtts / mL} = 21\text{ gtts / min}$

10. 563 mL

11. $\dfrac{50 \text{ mL}}{60 \text{ min}} \times 60 \text{ gtts} / \text{mL} = 50 \text{ gtts} / \text{min}$

12. $\dfrac{100 \text{ mL}}{60 \text{ min}} \times 10 \text{ gtts} / \text{mL} = 17 \text{ gtts} / \text{min}$. The answer is NO, because 20 gtts/min is too *fast*.

13. 400 mL (remaining)/50 = 8 hours

14. $\dfrac{500 \text{ mL}}{3 \times 60 \text{ min}} \times 15 \text{ gtts} / \text{mL} = 42 \text{ gtts} / \text{min}$

15. $\dfrac{250 \text{ mL}}{\text{x min}} \times 60 \text{ gtts} / \text{mL} = 125 \text{ gtts} / \text{min}$

    x = 120 min (or 2 h)

Exercise 7.3

1. Convert 42 lbs   = 19 kg
    first 10 kg   1 000 mL
    next 9 kg   450 mL   Total: 1 450 mL/day

2. Convert 12.25 lbs= 5.6 kg
    first 10 kg   560 mL   Total: 560 mL/day

3. first 10 kg   1 000 mL
    next 10 kg   500 mL
    remaining 30 kg   600 mL   Total: 2 100 mL/day

4. first 10 kg   1 000 mL
    next 10 kg   500 mL
    remaining 37 kg   740 mL   Total: 2 240 mL/day

5. 1 450/100 x 5 x 11.3 = 819 kj
6. 560/100 x 5 x 11.3 = 316 kj
7. 2 100/100 x 5 x 11.3 = 1 187 kj
8. 2 240/100 x 5 x 11.3 = 1 266 kj

Exercise 7.4

1. $\dfrac{1\,000 \text{ mL}}{10 \times 60 \text{ min}} \times 60 \text{ gtts} / \text{mL} = 100 \text{ gtts} / \text{min}$

2. IV rate = 100 gtts / min = $\dfrac{100}{60} = 1.7 \text{ mL} / \text{min}$

   $\dfrac{40 \text{ mmol}}{1\,000 \text{ mL}} = \dfrac{\text{x mmol}}{1.7 \text{ mL}} = 0.068 \text{ mmol per minute} = (0.07 \text{ mmol})$

3. $\dfrac{500 \text{ mL}}{10 \times 60 \text{ min}} \times 60 \text{ gtts} / \text{mL} = 50 \text{ gtts} / \text{min}$

4.   IV rate is $\dfrac{50 \text{ gtts / min}}{60 \text{ gtts / mL}} = 0.8 \text{ mL / min}$

$\dfrac{500 \text{ mg}}{500 \text{ mL}} = \dfrac{x \text{ mg}}{0.8 \text{ mL}} = 0.8$ mg of drug per minute

5.   Use 1 gram vial
6.   Add 9.5 mL sterile water to vial, shake well.
7.   Inspect solution in vial; if well mixed withdraw 10 mL, add to 1 litre bag of NS.

8. $\dfrac{1\,000 \text{ mL}}{12 \times 60 \text{ min}} \times 60 \text{ gtts / mL} = 83 \text{ gtts / min and } 83 \text{ mL / h}$

9.   Use within 24 h at room temperature and 72 hours under refrigeration.
10. 83 mL × 3 = 249 mL (approx): each mL contains 1 mg (1 g or 1 000 mg/1 000 mL) received approximately 249 (or 250) mg of drug.

Exercise 7.5

1. $\dfrac{200 \text{ mL}}{1 \times 60 \text{ min}} \times 60 \text{ gtts / mL} = 200 \text{ gtts / min}$

2.   500 mg:60 min = x mg:min
     x = 8.3 mg/min

3. $\dfrac{50 \text{ mL}}{30 \text{ min}} \times 60 \text{ gtts / mL} = 100 \text{ gtts / min}$

4.   250 mg:30 min = x mg:min
     x = 8.3 mg/min

5. $\dfrac{100 \text{ mL}}{60 \text{ min}} \times 60 \text{ gtts / mL} = 100 \text{ gtts / min}$

6.   500 mg/50 mL = 10 mg/mL
7.   125 mL:60 min = 100 mL:x mL. x = 48 minutes to infuse.
     Concentration: 5 000 units per mL
8.   Add 2 mL to minibag. Concentration: 1.6 mg/mL
9.   Although volume increases by 1 mL, not necessary to adjust.

     $\dfrac{50 \text{ mL}}{60 \text{ min}} \times 20 \text{ gtts / mL} = 17 \text{ gtts / min}$

10. Add 3.8 mL of sterile water for injection to 500 mg vial: shake well.
     Concentration is 125 mg/mL
11. Add 2 mL to 50 mL minibag. Concentration: 5 mg/mL

12. $\dfrac{100 \text{ mL}}{60 \text{ min}} \times 60 \text{ gtts / mL} = 100 \text{ gtts / min}$

13. 50 mL will infuse in 30 minutes = by 1330 h.
14. Add 2.5 mL to 1 000 mg vial and shake well.
15. Calculate: 334 mg:1 mL = 750 mg:x mL. x = 2.25 mL
     Add 2.25 mL to 100 mL minibag.

16. $\dfrac{100 \text{ mL}}{30 \text{ min}} \times 20 \text{ gtts / mL} = 67 \text{ gtts / min}$

17. $\dfrac{750 \text{ mg}}{100 \text{ mL}} = \dfrac{x \text{ mg}}{70 \text{ mL}}$ x = 525 mg

Exercise 7.6

1.   1 000 mg/50 mL = 20 mg/mL
2.   50 mL:x min = 100 mL:60 min. Infuse in 30 minutes

3. $\dfrac{50 \text{ mL}}{30 \text{ min}} \times 20 \text{ gtts / mL} = 33 \text{ gtts / min}$

4.   Add 10 mL sterile water
5.   If 1 g or 1 000 mg added to 25 mL = 40 mg/mL: cannot use
     If 1 g or 1 000 mg added to 50 mL = 20 mg/mL: can use

6. $\dfrac{50 \text{ mL}}{30 \text{ min}} \times 10 \text{ gtts / mL} = 17 \text{ gtts / min}$

7.   Label states slowly over 10-15 minutes.
8.   At 17 gtts/min x 20 min = 340 gtts.
     To convert to mL = 340/10 = 34 mL
     To determine drug infused: 1 000 mg:50 mL = x mg:34 mL. 680 mg absorbed.
9.   250 mg
10. 33 mL

Additional Practice

1. $\dfrac{50 \text{ mL}}{3 \times 60 \text{ min}} \times 10 \text{ gtts / mL} = 28 \text{ gtts / min}$

2.   60 min
3.   1330 h
4.   1 500 mL
5.   480 mL
6.   Use 2 vials. Add 20 mL sterile water, dissolve completely and add both vials.
7.   17 gtts/min
8.   63 x 2 = 126 mg of sodium
9.   Add to a 100 mL minibag
10. 33 gtts/min
11. 2.5 mg per mL
12. 125 gtts/min
13. 100 gtts/min (50 mL/30 min × 60)
14. 6 doses × 500 mg = 3 000 mg/24 h
15. Total = 2 925 mL (drug admin of 6 doses = 50 mL × 6 = 300 mL plus remaining 21 hours
     of IV infusing at 125 mL/h.

Case Study A

1.   NS for 3 doses (50 mL each) = 150 mL (time = 1.5 h)
2.   D5W for 2 doses (50 mL each) = 100 mL plus 21.5 hours @ 100 mL/h = 2 250 mL

3. 0600 - 0630 h   50 mL D5W (cefotetan dose)
    0630 - 0800 h   150 mL D5W (primary IV)
    0800 - 0830 h   50 mL NS (methylprednisolone dose)
    0830 - 1600 h   750 mL D5W (primary IV)
    1600 - 1630 h   50 mL NS (methylprednisolone dose)
    1630 - 1800 h   150 mL D5W (primary IV)
    1800 - 1830 h   50 mL D5W (cefotetan dose)
    1830 - 1900 h   50 mL D5W (primary IV)
    Total NS = 100 mL plus total D5W = 1 200 mL (Total IV fluid = 1 300 mL)

4. 2 doses cefotetan = 3 g and 2 doses methylprednisolone = 160 mg

5. (a) $\dfrac{100 \text{ mL}}{60 \text{ min}} \times 60 \text{ gtts} / \text{mL} = 100 \text{ gtts} / \text{min}$

    (b) $\dfrac{50 \text{ mL}}{30 \text{ min}} \times 60 \text{ gtts} / \text{mL} = 100 \text{ gtts} / \text{min}$

    (c) $\dfrac{50 \text{ mL}}{30 \text{ min}} \times 60 \text{ gtts} / \text{mL} = 100 \text{ gtts} / \text{min}$

Case Study B

1. new rate is 125 mL + 25 mL = 150 mL/h
2. new rate is 125 mL − 25 mL = 100 mL/h (reduce IV rate)
3. new rate is 125 mL/h (increase IV rate to original rate)

Postttest

1. $\dfrac{1\,000 \text{ mL}}{8 \times 60 \text{ min}} \times 60 \text{ gtts} / \text{mL} = 125 \text{ gtts} / \text{min}$

2. $\dfrac{1\,000 \text{ mL}}{8 \times 60 \text{ min}} \times 10 \text{ gtts} / \text{mL} = 21 \text{ gtts} / \text{min}$

3. 50 mL x 2 h = 100 mL

4. $\dfrac{100 \text{ mL}}{2 \times 60 \text{ min}} \times 60 \text{ gtts} / \text{mL} = 50 \text{ gtts} / \text{min}$

5. 25 mg of aminophylline

6. 10 hours

7. 50 mL of IV fluid (add 250 mg of drug to 50 mL of fluid to obtain concentration of 5 mg/mL).

8. $\dfrac{50 \text{ mL}}{30 \text{ min}} \times 60 \text{ gtts} / \text{mL} = 100 \text{ gtts} / \text{min}$

9. 375 mL should have been absorbed: 75 mL behind

10. $\dfrac{700 \text{ mL}}{5 \times 60 \text{ min}} \times 10 \text{ gtts} / \text{mL} = 23 \text{ gtts} / \text{min}$

Module 8

Exercise 8.1

1. Novolin ge NPH
2. slow acting
3. Novolin ge Lente
4. Slow acting
5. Humulin N
6. slow acting
7. 30 units/mL
8. 70 units/mL
9. 50 units/mL
10. 50 units/mL
11. 10 units/mL
12. 90 units/mL
13. 40 units/mL
14. 60 units/mL
15. 7 units regular and 7 units intermediate
16. 10 units regular and 40 units intermediate
17. 9 units regular and 21 units intermediate
18. 35 units regular and 35 units intermediate
19. 4 units regular and 36 units intermediate
20. 5 units regular and 20 units intermediate

Exercise 8.2

1. Regular (Product A)
2. NPH (Product B)
3. 18
4. NPH
5. 10
6. regular
7. 10
8. regular
9. 18
10. Lente
11. 28
12. Toronto (Product A)
13. NPH (Product B)
14. 26
15. NPH
16. 14
17. Toronto
18. 14
19. Toronto
20. 26
21. NPH
22. 40
23. Humulin R (Product E)
24. Humulin N (Product D)
25. 20
26. Humulin N
27. 10
28. Humulin R
29. 10
30. Humulin R
31. 20
32. Humulin N
33. 30
34. Humulin R (Product E)
35. Humulin N (Product D)
36. 11
37. Humulin N
38. 7
39. Humulin R
40. 7
41. Humulin R
42. 11
43. Humulin N
44. 18

Exercise 8.3

1. Use product (10 000 units/mL) Give 0.5 mL slowly IV.
2. 10 000:1 = 5 000:0.5 (5 000 = 5 000)
3. Use product (25 000 units/mL) Add 1 mL drug solution to 500 mL D5W.

    Convert 110 lbs = 50 kg
    Dose 20 units/kg/h = 1 000 units/h
    IV solution strength: 25 000 units/500 mL = 50 units/mL
    To deliver 1 000 units/h run IV at 20 mL/h. This is the base rate.

5. Increase rate by 6 mL = 26 mL/h
6. 26 mL × 50 units/mL = 1 300 units/h
7. Increase rate by 3 mL/h = 29 mL/h
8. 29 mL × 50 units/mL = 1 450 units/h
9. 0915 - 1315 (4 h) rate @ 20 mL/h = 80 mL
    1315 - 1915 (6 h) rate @ 26 mL/h = 156 mL
    1915 - 2315 (4 h) @ 29 mL/h = 116 mL
    TOTAL: 352 mL
10. bolus of 5 000 units
    0915 - 1315 (4 h) heparin rate of 1 000 units/h = 4 000 units
    1315 - 1915 (6 h) heparin rate of 1 300 units/h = 7 800 units
    1915 - 0915 (14 h) heparin rate of 1 450 units/h = 20 300 units
    TOTAL: 37 100 units

Case Study #1

A.
Lasix (1) 60 mg (odd day); (2) give 1-40 mg and 1-20 mg tablet of furosemide (Lasix).
morphine (3) 300 mg; (4) give 1 tab 300 mg MS Contin
levothyroxine sodium (5) 0.1 mg (6) use Synthroid 0.1 mg and give 1 tab

B.
7. 600 mg plus any for breakthrough pain
8. give 1 tab of morphine 30 mg
9. use literature, examine for any markings, compare with drug supply, call pharmacy
10. no: should receive 60 mg on odd days.

Case Study #2

Drug name	Drug ordered	Product used	Amount given
(1) Procan SR	(2) 750 mg PO	(3) A	(4) 1 tab
(5) Cardizem	(6) 60 mg PO	(7) F	(8) 1 tab
(9) Lasix	(10) 40 mg PO	(11) H	(12) 1 tab

Case Study #3

1. docusate sodium
2. capsule
3. 100 mg per cap
4. 2 caps
5. 0830 h
6. 1600 h
5. 0830 h
6. 1600 h
7. yes (1–12 g daily in divided doses q8–12h)

8. Use label B. Vial of 2 g. Add 20 mL of sterile water for injection. Shake well.
9. 95 mg ceftizoxime per mL
10. Add entire contents of vial (approximately 21.4 mL)
11. Note: added approx 21.4 mL to a 50 mL minibag: concentration is 2 g/71.4 mL or approx 28 mg/mL (This is a good situation to use a reconstitution device. Total volume would be controlled)
12. 24 h room temp, 48 h refrigerator
13. 0930 h (approx)
14. 1700 h
15. @ 100 mL/h = 2 400 mL
16. 2 250 mL NS
17. 3 doses of 50 mL = 150 mL D5W
18. Add 3 mL sterile water or bacteriostatic water for inj. Shake well
19. 270 mg ceftizoxime per mL
20. 3.7 mL IM
21. Add 6 mL sterile or bacteriostatic water for injection
22. 3.7 mL IM
23. 24 h room temp, 48 h refrigerator
24. 2 doses (3.7 mL each)

Case Study #4: Medications for several patients

M.A.R. Mr. Ziebart   0800 h
Order   **Number of tablets**
(1) Capoten 12.5 mg   (2) F   (3) 1/2 tab (25 mg tab)
(4) Lasix 20 mg   (5) H   (6) 1 tab (20 mg tab)
(7) Atasol 15   (8) I   (9) 1 tab

M.A.R. Mrs. Flanagan   0800h
Order   **Number of tablets**
(10) Desyrel 50 mg   (11) M   (12) 1 tab (50 mg tab)
(13) digoxin 0.375 mg   (14) J and K   (15) 1 tab (250 mcg) plus
     1 tab (0.125 mg)
     or give 3 tabs of 0.125 mg
(16) lorazepam 0.5 mg   (17) N   (18) 1 tab (0.5 mg tab)
(19) Entrophen 500 mg   (20) B   (21) 1 tab (0.5 g tab)
(22) Cytotec 0.1 mg   (23) G   (24) 1 tab (100 mcg)

M.A.R. Miss Perman   0800 h
Order   **Number of tablets**
(25) Simemet 100/10   (26) C   (27) 1 tab (100/10)
   and 250   (26) D   plus 1 tab (250)
(28) digoxin 0.25 mg   (29) J   (30) 1 tab (250 mcg)

Case Study #5

1. To provide 5 mg/h: 200 mg : 500 mL = 5 mg : x mL x = (12.5) 13mL/h
2. To provide 6 mg/h: 200 mg : 500 mL = 6 mg : x mL x = 15 mL/h
3. To provide 7 mg/h: 200 mg : 500 mL = 7 mg : x mL x = (17.5) 18 mL/h
4. To provide 8 mg/h: 200 mg : 500 mL = 8 mg : x mL x = 20 mL/h

5.   Total dose: 65.25 mg of morphine

Time	Vehicle	Dosage
2300-0115 (2.25 h)	IV 5 mg/h	11.25 mg
0115	IM	5 mg
0115-0345 (2.5 h)	IV 6 mg/h	15 mg
0345	IM	5 mg
0345-0545 (2 h)	IV 7 mg/h	14 mg
0545	IM	5 mg
0545-0700 h (1.25 h)	IV 8 mg/h	10 mg

Case Study #6

1.   0 units
2.   10 units
3.   5 units
4.   0 units
5.   0 units
6.   8 units
7.   5 units
8.   0
9.   10 units
10.   15 units on day 1
     13 units on day 2

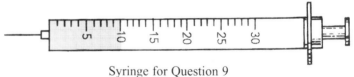

Syringe for Question 9

Module 9

Exercise 9.1

1.   4 mg/kg/day = 4 × 20 = 80 mg daily
2.   80 mg/4 = 20 mg each dose
3.   5 mg/kg/day = 5 × 51.2 = 256 mg/day
4.   Yes, not to exceed 400 mg daily
5.   Daily dose is 345 mg × 4 doses = 1 380 mg/day
6.   Range is 20 mg/kg/dose, 20 × 34.5 = 690 to 50 mg/kg, 50 × 34.5 = 1 725 mg.
     Yes, 1 380 is within the range.
7.   125 mg:5 mL = 345 mg:x mL   x = 13.8 mL (or 14 mL)
8.   Range is 10-15 mg/kg each dose = (10 × 22.5) = 225 mg to (15 × 22.5) = 327.5 mg/dose
9.   Jennifer is 10 years old. 325-650 mg each dose is the appropriate range.
     Yes, 480 is within the range.
10.   Range is (10 × 12.6) = 126 mg to (15 × 12.6) = 189 mg.
     Dose is too low and may not be effective.
11.   160 mg:5 mL = 170 mg:x mL   x = 5.3 mL

12. Convert 13 lbs = 5.9 kg
Limit range (0.015 × 5.9) = 0.0885 to (0.035 × 5.9) = 0.2065 mg
Convert to mcg 88.5 to 206.5, so dose of 175 mcg is within range.
13. 250 mcg:1 mL = 175 mcg:x mL   x = 0.7 mL
14. 25% of 175 mcg = 43.75 mcg
50 mcg:1 mL = 43.75 mcg:x mL   x = 0.875 mL or 1 mL (oral)
15. Range (0.5 × 17) = 8.5 mg to (1 × 17) = 17 mg. Yes the dose is within the range.
16. 20 mg:1 mL = 8.5 mg:x mL   x = 0.425 mL = 0.43 mL
17. 8.5 × 4 = 34 mg
18. Recommended dose is 0.01 mL × 1mg/ml = 0.01 mg. Convert to mcg = 0.01 × 1 000 mcg/mL = 10 mcg/kg. Yes the dose is within range.
19. Lara's dose is 10 mcg × 15 kg = 150 mcg. Solution is 1 mg/mL or 1 000 mcg/mL.
1 000 mcg: 1 mL = 150 mcg: x mL   x = 0.15 mL
20.

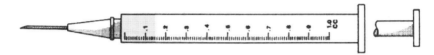

Exercise 9.2

1. 5 mg × 17 kg = 85 mg/dose
25 mg:1 mL = 85 mg:x mL   x = 3.4 mL = 3 mL
2. 5 mg × 11.5 kg = 57.5 mg/dose
125 mg:5 mL = 57.5 mg:x mL   x = 2.3 mL = 2 mL
3. 0.015 mg × 3.2 kg = 0.048 mg
0.25 mg:1 mL = 0.048 mg:x mL   x = 0.192 mL = 0.19 mL
4. 0.01 mg × 34 kg = 0.34 mg; Yes this dosage is safe.
5. Convert 19 lbs = 8.6 kg
2 mg × 8.6 kg = 17.2
15 mg:5 mL = 17.2 mg:x mL   x = 5.73 mL = 6 mL
6. 2 mg × 3.9 kg = 7.8 mg
10 mg:1 mL = 7.8 mg:x mL   x = 0.78 mL
7. 20 mg:2 mL = 2 mg:x mL   x = 0.2 mL
8. 50 mg × 11.2 kg ÷ 4 doses = 140 mg/dose
125 mg:1 mL = 140 mg:x mL   x = 1.12 mL
9. Convert 860 g = 0.86 kg
Dose = 0.6 mg × 0.86 kg ÷ 6 doses = 0.09 mg
Give 2 mg: 1 mL = 0.09 mg: x mL   x = 0.045 or 0.05 mL
10. Received 60 mg × 6 doses = 360 mg
Max is 65 mg × 7.2 kg = 468 mg. This dose has not exceeded the limit.

Pediatric Case Study

1. q8h or tid
2. 115 mg
3. 0.9 mL
4. 3.8 mL diluent added to 500 mg vial
5. Convert 32 lbs = 14.5 kg; 25 mg × 14.5 = 363.75 mg daily

6. 3 equal doses = 121.5 mg each dose
7. 115 mg compare to 121 mg: explanation – table uses approximations
8. Each dose 85 mg; give 0.7 mL

Exercise 9.3

1. Convert 600 g = 0.6 kg; dose 2.5 mg × 0.6 kg = 1.5 mg. Add 0.15 mL
2. Convert 11 lbs = 5 kg; 7.5 mg × 5 kg = 37.5 mg by IV infusion
3. Add 25 mg. Available 50 mg/5 mL = add 2.5 mL to 25 mL minibag.
4. Dose required = 0.5 mg × 5 kg = 2.5 mg/h = 2.5 mL/h
5. 2 mcg × 1.265 kg × 60 min = 151.8 mcg/h
6. 5 mcg × 0.79 kg × 60 min × 50 mL = 11 850 mcg
   11 850 mcg / 40 000 mcg = 0.296 (0.3) mL
7. 1 mL/h
8. Rate is 0.5 mL/h
9. 7.5 mcg × 1.17 kg × 60 min × 50 mL = 26 325 mcg
   26 325 mcg/40 000 mcg = 0.66 mL
10. 7.5 mcg × 1.17 kg × 60 min = 526.5 mcg per h

Exercise 9.4

1. $\dfrac{3 \text{ mcg} \times 52 \text{ kg} \times 60 \text{ min}}{400 \text{ mcg} / \text{mL}} = (23.4)$ or, 23 mL / h

2. $\dfrac{4 \text{ mcg} \times 64 \text{ kg} \times 60 \text{ min}}{400 \text{ mcg} / \text{mL}} = (38.4)$ or, 38 mL / h

3. $\dfrac{6 \text{ mcg} \times 77 \text{ kg} \times 60 \text{ min}}{400 \text{ mcg} / \text{mL}} = (69.3)$ or, 69 mL / h

4. $\dfrac{5 \text{ mcg} \times 75 \text{ kg} \times 60 \text{ min}}{400 \text{ mcg} / \text{mL}} = (56.25)$ or, 56 mL / h

5. Convert 178 lbs = 81 kg

   $\dfrac{8 \text{ mcg} \times 81 \text{ kg} \times 60 \text{ min}}{400 \text{ mcg} / \text{mL}} = (97.2)$ or, 97 mL / h

Exercise 9.5

1. 400 mg = 400 × 1 000 = 400 000 mcg/500 mL = 800 mcg/mL
2. 250 mg = 250 × 1 000 = 250 000 mcg/250 mL = 1 000 mcg/mL
3. 1 mg = 1 000 mcg/250 mL = 4 mcg/mL

   $\dfrac{3.5 \text{ mcg} \times 60 \text{ min}}{4 \text{ mcg} / \text{mL}} = 52.5$ or 53 mL / h

4. Concentration = 200 mg (200 000 mcg in 250 mL = 800 mcg/mL)

   $\dfrac{3 \text{ mcg} \times 70 \text{ kg} \times 60 \text{ min}}{800 \text{ mcg} / \text{mL}} = (15.75)$ or, 16 mL / h

5.   2 mcg × 65 kg = 130 mcg per minute: In 1 h = 130 × 60 = 7 800 mcg
6.   200 mg (200 000 mcg) in 250 mL = 800 mcg per mL
7.   800 mcg:1 mL = 7 800:x mL   x = (9.75) or, 10 mL/h
8.   1 mg = 1 000 mcg/250 mL = 4 mcg per mL
9.   50 mg:250 mL = x mg:60 mL   x = 12 mg/h = 12/60 = 0.2 mg or 200 mcg/min
10.   (a) 1 mg   (b) 30 mL/h   (c) 3 mcg/min × 15 = 45 mcg
11.   (a) 8 mcg/mL   (b) 8 ml/h   (c) 3 mcg/min
12.   (a) 1 mcg/min   (b) 45 mL/h   (c) 2 × 30 = 60 mcg
    (d) NO should be 60 mL/h (e) 1 mg/250 mL = x mg/200 mL = 0.8 mg or 800 mcg

Case Studies

1.   give 5 mL of 20 mg/mL strength
2.   Add 2 g to 500 mL bag (use 2, 50 mL vials)
3.   Run at 60 mL/h
4.   Use 2, 5 mL ampules (10 mL = 1 000 mg)
5.   Add 2 g (4, 5 mL ampules) to 500 mL
6.   Infuse at 60 gtts/min
7.   Add 2 g (2, 50 mL vials) to 500 mL: infuse at 15 mL/h
8.   Give 2 mL of 10 mg/mL strength
9.   Add 2 mg (or 2, 5 mL ampules) to 500 mL; infuse at 30 gtts/min
10.   2 mcg/min = 30 gtts/min and 3 mcg/min = 45 gtts/min
    2.5 mcg/min is midway between 30 and 45 = 37.5 (or 38) gtts/min

Posttest

1.   875 mg
2.   Yes: this dose is within recommended range: 15 kg × 6 mg/kg = 90 mg
                                    15 kg × 12 mg/kg = 180 mg
3.   No: it is lower than the recommended dosage of 1 050 daily
4.   3 tablets
5.   dose = 20 mcg× 50 kg = 100 mcg. Give 0.25 mL
6.   2 mg × 70 kg = 140 mg. Give 0.9 mL
7.   0.315 = 0.32 mg
8.   0.8 mL
9.   650 mg per dose
10.   0.55 mL
11.   126 mcg/minute
12. $\dfrac{2 \text{ mcg} \times 60 \text{ kg} \times 60 \text{ min}}{1\,000 \text{ mcg}/\text{mL}} = 7 \text{ mL}/\text{h or } 7 \text{ gtts}/\text{min}$
13.   80 mg/100 mL = 800 mcg per mL
    15 gtts/min = 15 mL/h = 15/60 = 0.25 mL per min
    800 × 0.25 = 200 mcg/min
14.   0.3 mg × 33 kg = 9.9 mg: received 10 mg; dose is not correct, however in emergency situations quick action is required and the error of 0.1 mg may not be significant.
15.   10 × 21.2 = 212 mg/4 doses = 53 mg per dose
16.   0.78 mL
17.   3.9 mL
18.   237 mcg/min
19.   14 gtts/min or 14 mL/h
20   17 gtts/min or 17 mL/h

Index

RULES FOR ARITHMETIC OF FRACTIONS

To add fractions: find the common denominator; convert each fraction to an equivalent fraction using the common denominator; add the numerators; place the sum over the denominator; simplify.

To subtract fractions: find the common denominator; convert each fraction to an equivalent fraction using the common denominator; subtract the numerators; place the sum over the denominator; simplify.

To multiply fractions: multiply the numerators; multiply the denominators; place the product of the numerators over the product of the denominators; simplify.

To divide fractions: invert the terms of the divisor (the number that is being divided into the dividend); use multiplication of fractions.

To simplify a fraction: divide the numerator and denominator by the same number.

RULES FOR ARITHMETIC OF MIXED NUMBERS

To add mixed numbers: add the whole numbers; add the fractions and simplify if necessary; combine the two sums.

To subtract mixed numbers: subtract the whole numbers — or convert the mixed numbers to improper fractions; subtract the fractions and simplify if necessary.

To multiply mixed numbers: express the mixed number as an improper fraction and proceed as for multiplication of fractions.

To divide mixed numbers: express the mixed number as an improper fraction and proceed as for division of fractions.